Ethical Issues in Nursing

a proceedings

Adapted from Nursing Institutes
held in Boston, Chicago, Houston
and San Francisco during 1975-76
and sponsored by

School of Nursing
Catholic University of America
Washington, D.C.

and

Department of Nursing Services
The Catholic Hospital Association
St. Louis, Missouri

THE CATHOLIC HOSPITAL ASSOCIATION
St. Louis, Missouri 63104

Library of Congress Catalog Card No. 76-24218
ISBN 0-87125-033-0

Introduction

The tremendous expansion of scientific knowledge and the development of sophisticated technologies in the health care field have given rise to questions concerning life, death, and Christian values. Registered nurses and nursing students, ill-informed on ethical issues, experience conflicts of conscience because of clinical problems they encounter in various secular or denominational health care facilities. Consequently, administrators of health care facilities and others concerned about ethical issues have requested that such ethical issues be clarified. As a result of such requests, officials of The Catholic Hospital Association and the Catholic University of America developed and co-sponsored four institutes on Ethical Issues in Nursing.

The contents of this manual are adapted from the papers presented by speakers at the four institutes. We are deeply grateful to the speakers who were so generous in working with us throughout the past year. In editing their papers for this publication, some of the personal experiences had to be deleted. The information exchanged during lively discussion periods has also been excluded.

For those who attended, but more especially for those who were unable to be present, we hope that this publication will serve as a springboard for exploration of the crucial ethical issues facing nurses today. While there may not be definite answers to all of these issues, nurses may be consoled in knowing that their questions are of concern to others. These questions are not exclusively nursing issues. Rather, they are ethical issues affecting every Christian and cannot be ignored.

Sister Elaine Catellier, DC
Director of Nursing Services
The Catholic Hospital Association

Contents

A Christian View of Sickness and Suffering

FRANCIS X. CLEARY, SJ

To consider sickness and suffering from a Judeo-Christian point of view is to reflect upon suffering as essentially a mystery. This means that suffering is incapable of an explanation in terms fully comprehensible to the human mind. In the Old Testament, God responded to Job's demand for an explanation of suffering and death by saying, in effect, "I couldn't tell you, even if I wanted to; I would like to, but you cannot understand."

Suffering, however, is not the only mystery; life, disease, death, and the human person are all mysterious in that they are incapable of complete explanation. And merely because suffering is a mystery does not mean that we are unable to come to a fuller (if not complete) understanding of this reality. Because suffering is an essential part of the human experience, we must probe for insights into it and for a better understanding of that which will never be fully comprehended.

I am interested in presenting the Judeo-Christian teaching on suffering because such an approach is probably shared by a large number of patients and practitioners, and because the Judeo-Christian tradition contains valuable insights even for those who do not share a commitment to this tradition.

In conformity with the Judeo-Christian revelation on suffering, I would like to discuss three main points, each one of which is essential and all of which are interrelated. First, in the Judeo-Christian tradition, suffering is *real*. Thus, it is opposed to a position such as the Christian Science attitude which denies the reality of suffering by asserting that the idea of suffering exists only in the mind and can be eradicated. For these people, only the mind is real and nothing physical should be allowed to bother us.

But the Judeo-Christian teaches that suffering is real and that it is *evil*. Thus, this tradition is also opposed to the kind of pious idealism which looks upon suffering as a thing to be desired. In the New Testament, Jesus never confronts suffering by saying to the afflicted person, "This is good for you; offer it up." Rather, when he

1

encounters sickness, Jesus invariably is concerned with healing. He can't always cure, because no one can be cured by Jesus unless he wants to be, unless he opens himself in trust to the healing power of God. Thus we see that suffering is both real and evil, and that pious idealizing of suffering is fundamentally opposed to the Judeo-Christian tradition.

But if suffering is real and evil, how can we explain it? If it is evil, how can it come from God? When we confront authentic Judeo-Christian revelation about God, we find a Being who is radically loving, accepting, forgiving, and long-suffering — a God whose love is limitless. This is very important, because the basic point of Judeo-Christian revelation is who God is, what He is like. The images of God used in the Bible are intent upon explaining, in language we can comprehend, what God, so wholly and completely other, is like. Thus God reveals Himself as a loving Father in Hosea 11:1-9, a Father so completely caught up in His Love for His little child that the child is everything for Him. We can understand this image. We've all seen the example of a young man who lives a pleasant, carefree life but who, upon marriage and becoming a father, gives up his youthful diversions because his child means more to him than such things as a car or a boat. His world is now summed up in that little child who he carries around in his arms. And God uses this image to talk about himself in relationship to us.

In the first three chapters of Hosea, God presents an even more powerful image of Himself. In telling about the fidelity of Hosea's love for a wife who has wronged him by running off with other men, he shows Himself to be a constant lover who forgives the wrongs done Him by those He loves with tenderness and reconciliation.

Likewise, in the New Testament, God reveals Himself in the image of a friend. Jesus was a friend to all — publicans as well as the God-fearing, prostitutes as well as the pious. And the quality of His friendship was radically open. He didn't go around accusing or damning or condemning. His love was non-judgmental and accepting. He cursed nobody; He punished nobody; He loved everybody.

These Old and New Teatament images of God reveal Him to be all-good and all-loving. But this concept of God creates a real problem when we try to reconcile it with the fact of suffering. Since suffering is a real evil, it cannot be caused by a good and loving God.

Whence, then, does suffering come? According to Judeo-Christian revelation, all suffering is somehow associated with or caused by human *sin*. This is a basic article of Judeo-Christian revelation and faith. Suffering is caused not by God, but by my personal and our corporate sins. Anything that is evil and destructive in the world owes its origin not to the God who wanted to create a perfect universe, but to human sin which from the beginning frustrated

God's design and caused the kind of situation in which there is both good and evil, including all suffering.

There are times when we can show that a concrete example of suffering is directly caused by a particular sin. If we wake up one morning with a hangover, we can directly relate our suffering to intemperate drinking. But the question is: Can we analyze every instance of suffering in that way? Obviously not. This situation is brought out very well in Chapter IX of the Gospel of John. Upon seeing a young man who was obviously blind from birth, the disciples asked their teacher: "Who sinned — he or his parents?" Jesus replied that the blindness was caused neither by his own sin nor by sins of his parents. Rather, he leaves the impression that it is the sin of the whole human race that causes such suffering. In other words, this kind of evil is the whole meaning of the story of the first parents' sin. In God's original plan, there would be no suffering because there would be no death and everybody would live in a totally non-exploitative, non-violent way. But from the very beginning this plan was frustrated by human sin. Thus, suffering is caused by human sin, and each person who is born approves and ratifies that original sin by his or her own sins.

Nor is sin something that a person can do and then walk away from. Its effects radiate out in ever-widening circles. By sinning, we introduce evil into the world, and one act of sinful unloving has profound consequences that cannot be blotted out. Such is the power and permanence of evil.

This reflection on the origin of suffering leads us to the third point: If God is good, how can He *allow* sin and thus suffering to exist in the world? The answer is this: God, who is all-good and all-loving, can permit suffering *only* because a greater good can be obtained as a result of suffering than without it. In other words, God allows suffering only insofar as it contains the potential for becoming the privileged means of growth and love. What does it mean to allow suffering? Suffering is permitted to exist not merely because it is an opportunity to learn from our mistakes, but because at its deepest level it is the best way to grow in love.

Let me give an example of what I mean about growing in love through suffering. Some years ago, an older Jesuit priest involved himself with a minority group in St. Louis. He lived their life style, ate their kind of food, gave himself totally to whatever they needed that he as a Catholic priest could to do for them. The people whom he had come to help were grateful, of course, but they were not sure about his motives. Was he doing this because he loved them, or because he had a guilt complex, or because he just wanted something to do in his later years?

One day he took some children on a picnic. They rented a couple of canoes, and a little girl who couldn't swim fell overboard. Although he too couldn't swim, he jumped out of the boat. For a split second, he had the choice of grabbing onto the canoe himself or holding up the girl to be rescued. He chose to save the girl and, as a result, he drowned. The funeral was very moving. The minority group attended in force — young and old, male and female. There was a certain sense of sadness in their behavior, but the overriding emotion was joy. They were joyful because *now they knew:* This man had really loved them. In the face of death, they had seen an unambiguous expression of love — by dying he proved his love. He made his greatest act of love in that moment when he chose to save the child. I think this capsulizes the whole meaning of suffering in terms of the Judeo-Christian tradition. Suffering is evil and is never going to be anything other than evil, but it has a tremendous potential for becoming the means of growth in love.

Why did the suffering and death of Jesus Christ redeem all humankind? Because God is a sadist who refused to forgive unless somebody suffered? No, that's absurd. God could not accept Jesus' suffering and death as something pleasing in itself. And Jesus' attitude in the garden the night before his death was sound and mentally healthy: I don't want it; it's evil; nevertheless, not my will but yours be done. Jesus' death on the cross was evil, but at the same time it was His supreme expression of love. And that is the reason why we are redeemed: By His love, rather than merely by the pain He endured.

As Christians, therefore, we cannot be complacent in our attitude toward suffering. We cannot just shrug it off and say, "That's the way life is." As long as any person is suffering, I, as a Christian, must be radically discontented. I am obligated to do everything I can to mitigate the suffering and pray to God to hasten the coming of the Kingdom when all suffering will be eliminated. The Judeo-Christian tradition is dedicated to the total elimination of suffering.

On the other hand, in the face of suffering, anguish, and pain, the true Christian cannot shake his fist at God and place the blame on Him. All he can do is look into himself and say that it is his sinfulness, his unwillingness to love, that has caused a universe in which pain and suffering exist. We cannot blame suffering on God. Rather we must blame ourselves, our own infidelity, our own inability to love selflessly.

Finally, let us consider the individual person who is undergoing suffering, who is being presented with an opportunity for growth and self-acceptance and maturity. I think the important thing to remember is that people who are dying (especially tragic deaths, such as young mothers dying of cancer) want desperately that their suffering and death be meaningful. They don't want to waste it. How can this be achieved?

One way is for those of us who have witnessed this suffering to become better as a result. We can be inspired by their example of patient acceptance of that which cannot be resisted. We can become more sensitive, more loving of the life that we have, and more willing to share and give than we had been previously. This kind of suffering and death has great potential for growth in love if we, the larger human community, allow it to function as it can. Suffering can have meaning and enduring value if we allow it to become part of the redemptive work of Christ — the victory of love through suffering.

The world is like a river. At one end we are pumping in pollutants — evil and sin. At the other end, we have a filter plant taking the pollutants out. Pumped in by our unlovingness, these pollutants can be removed by our acceptance of the kind of suffering we can't get rid of as a means of neutralizing some of the evil. In this way, the redemption begun in Jesus Christ continues into and permeates our own lives.

What is Ethics?

LEONARD J. WEBER, PhD

To understand ethical problems today and effectively deal with them requires an understanding of diverse ethical orientations. Since most people we come into contact with have been influenced more by contemporary culture than by traditional Catholic teaching, it is imperative for us to know something about the various ethical approaches and how the Catholic approach compares and contrasts with these others.

Part I — Some Common Mistakes

One of the most common mistakes that is made in attempting to satisfactorily solve ethical problems is to identify morality with practicality. It is interesting to note how the notion of practicality works in day-to-day discussions of ethical questions. What is sought is the greatest good for the greatest number. Those who see morality in terms of practicality approach ethics in the context of the possible benefits to society and emphasize those benefits that are material or tangible. Joseph Fletcher, a prominent Christian proponent of a type of situation ethics, is dedicated to the ethics of practicality. I would like to borrow from Fletcher one example of the practical approach to ethical problem-solving. He presents the case of a woman who underwent amniocentesis during her first pregnancy and was told that her fetus had the deadly Tay-Sachs disease. Consequently, she had an abortion. After being told that she and her husband had a one-in-four chance of each of their children being affected with Tay-Sachs, she was asked whether she thought it might be better not to conceive again. " 'No,' she answered, 'I will conceive again and again and again, if necessary, and I will abort and abort, until a sound and healthy child comes to us.' That is what happened. Not until the fourth pregnancy did the disease fail to show up, and then a normal son was born. . . ."[1] To Fletcher, this was a good decision because the woman made certain, as far as she was able, that she had a healthy child. She was concerned about the consequences, that neither the child, the parents, nor society would have to suffer. As a result, she took whatever steps were necessary to achieve that goal. She was practical.

Besides Fletcher, there are other representatives of the practicality

6

ethic. Garrett Hardin, a well-known biologist, reflecting on the problems of world food shortage, overpopulation, and the relationship of the rich nations to the poor nations, has formulated what he calls "lifeboat ethics." He writes: "Metaphorically, each rich nation amounts to a lifeboat full of comparatively rich people. The poor of the world are in other, much more crowded lifeboats. Continuously, so to speak, the poor fall out of their lifeboats and swim for a while in the water outside, hoping to be admitted to a rich lifeboat, or in some other way to benefit from the 'goodies' on board. What should the passengers in the rich lifeboat do?"[2] Hardin answers the question with a long analysis which allegedly shows that whatever is done to help the poor of the world will be too little to save them but enough to weaken our own chances for survival. To be really practical, we should abandon the poor nations to their starvation so that at least the rich nations can survive. Otherwise, we are not serving posterity.

The greatest good for the greatest number is here interpreted in terms of the future. As Hardin argues, "Every life saved this year in a poor country diminishes the quality of life for subsequent generations."[3] It is simply not practical — not in the interest of the race as a whole — to act with generosity toward those less fortunate.

Another guise under which morality is sometimes hidden — though not quite so dramatic as practicality — effectively makes ethical questions look different from what they really are. This is morality seen as opinion. The Roman statesman Cicero wrote in *De Legibus* (I. 17, 45): "Only a madman could maintain that the distinction between the honorable and the dishonorable, between virtue and vice, is a matter of opinion, not of nature." But this is exactly what the contention of this second wrong approach is: Right or wrong has nothing to do with nature or with facts, but is merely a matter of opinion.

The identification of morality as opinion may be one of the consequences of the scientific age, a logical result of the emphasis on the scientific method. Fact has come to be understood as that which is empirically verifiable. And, unfortunately, truth has often become identified with and limited to fact. Thus, anything that is not verifiable is neither factual nor true; it is merely an opinion or a value judgment. Consequently, ethical principles or moral stands, since they are not facts, are merely opinions and are no more important than tastes or prejudices or arbitrary choices.

It is easy to see how the notion of opinion can sidetrack ethical discussions. Whereas, practicality attempts to translate all ethical questions into calculations of benefit for society, opinion reduces all ethical questions to expressions of personal likes and dislikes.

One of the primary expressions of this approach to ethics is what I sometimes call the Tolerance Ethic. The Tolerance Ethic is expressed

7

in statements like these: "I know what I think is right, but I cannot tell someone else what is right for him or her;" "I don't want to impose my opinion on someone else;" "The most important thing is that everyone be left free to decide for himself or herself what is right." Because morality is seen as merely a matter of opinion, the most important concern is the determination not to impose a position on someone else. We might agree that tastes are unique to the individual and not to be imposed. The Tolerance Ethic goes a step further and says the same thing about morality: Just because I think abortion is wrong is no reason to tell you that it would be wrong for you to have an abortion.

It is not easy to give examples of the Tolerance Ethic at work. On every question it takes pretty much the same stand; namely, that I cannot tell you what is the right or wrong thing for you to do. The Tolerance Ethic was behind many of the moves to legalize abortion, using the argument that the law should not be used to impose the opinion of some on those who disagree. Much of the opposition to possible anti-abortion amendments to the Constitution takes the same approach, viewing abortion as a question of the freedom of opinion or the freedom of religion.

The approach to morality as opinion makes it very difficult, if not impossible, to set limits to what is morally acceptable. Paul Ramsey suggests that the moral thinking of many people will lead them to condone the action taken in this hypothetical case: A 42-year-old widower had only one child, a 15-year-old son who was dying of a heart condition. The father feels that he has had some opportunity for life while his son has not. He decides he would like to sacrifice his life for his son by donating his healthy heart to replace his son's inadequate one. He finds a surgeon who is willing to perform the operation. The father and son (the son knows nothing about who the donor is) are both taken to the operating room. The father is placed under general anesthesia and the transfer of the heart takes place.[4]

Morality as opinion can and does lead to a justification of this type of procedure. Since we can in no way prove that it is morally wrong to kill oneself for someone else, do we have the right to refuse to let this man carry out his wishes? If we don't let him do what he thinks is right, we are imposing our opinions on him.

The morality of opinion approach does not feel a need to justify moral stands that are being taken. If morality is merely a matter of opinion, there is no need for me to explain to you (or perhaps even to myself) why I am doing what I am doing. Whether my decision is arbitrary or well thought out makes little difference. What makes it right is that it is *my* opinion. With a full emphasis on individual opinion, rational discussion of moral issues comes to an end.

In addition to morality as practicality and morality as opinion, there is one more way in which morality is disguised; namely, subjectivity. Morality as subjectivity is an extreme version of a legitimate and serious effort to recognize the importance of attitudes in morality.

The extreme emphasis on subjectivity translates all discussions of morality into discussions of motive or intention or attitude. An act is good if it is done in the right spirit or with the right purpose, so that whatever is done lovingly is good and whatever is done with malice is evil. To lie out of a spirit of love is good; to lie out of a desire to hurt is evil. To have an abortion as an expression of one's loving concern for the child is good; to have an abortion to spite one's husband is evil. And so on.

The focus on the intention or the motive as being most important in determining morality greatly reduces the need to carefully distinguish between different types of actions. In the euthanasia controversy, for example, those who emphasize the importance of motive or intention see little or no difference between letting someone die by withholding extraordinary treatment and directly intervening to bring about the death. In both cases, the intention is to try to achieve as good a death as possible under the circumstances. In both cases, the decision is motivated by concern for the dying patient. According to this type of moral thinking, there is no moral difference between the two types of actions.

Subjectivity is, of course, a close relative of opinion. If something is moral or not depending upon the subjective attitude, then morality depends upon the individual situation. This approach involves the same kind of individualism and denial of objective morality as does the opinion approach. The understanding of morality as subjectivity also supports the Tolerance Ethic. I cannot tell you what is right and you cannot tell me, because we don't know each other's attitudes and motives.

Traditionally, a distinction has been made between objective morality and subjective morality. Objective morality has to do with the morality of the *action*, with *what* is being done. Subjective morality has to do with the interior dimension — with the attitudes and the motives of the person performing the action. Traditionally, there has been a reluctance to judge someone's subjective morality. The question of whether or not an individual is following his own best conscience can appropriately be left to that person and to God. What we must concern ourselves with is objective morality. We must make sure that our consciences are properly formed regarding what is and is not good behavior, and we must do our part in helping others form their consciences. Here we must, in a sense, render judgment. We need to tell others what is right and what is wrong. But such judgment or advice or criticism is not a judgment of the other person's motives or attitudes. It is merely a judgment of behavior.

9

On the basis of this traditional distinction between objective and subjective morality, it is easy to see what happens when morality is defined almost exclusively in terms of subjectivity. It reduces behavior to something that is so private, so individualistic that we hesitate to say anything about it except to urge good intentions. As in the case of morality as opinion, morality as subjectivity renders all rational discussion of ethics nearly meaningless.

These are three of the paths that are often taken in moral thinking in our contemporary culture. The first path — practicality — leads to the resolution of ethical questions in terms of our perceived material welfare. The second path — opinion — does not lead to any particular solution of ethical questions, but merely allows each person to go his own way. The third path — subjectivity — leads to the resolution of all moral questions in terms of attitude and motivation. Those who travel the second and third paths often arrive at the Tolerance Ethic as their final destination.

I present the three approaches described above not so that you may choose one of them but so that you may recognize what must be avoided. None of these approaches is profitable, and none leads to a true resolution of ethical dilemmas. Each one is destructive of true morality. The first denies that there are any moral limits to what may be done, because anything may be perpetrated in the name of the greatest good for the greatest number. The second denies that there is any such thing as morality at all, because it does not provide a basis for determining whether any action is inherently good or evil. The third approach leads to the same type of danger and the same failure to provide guidelines. With a good motive anything is acceptable, no matter what. There is a very basic flaw that is common to all three of these approaches.

Part II — Two Ethical Worldviews

On the one hand, there are the three misguided approaches to ethical thinking that I have discussed above. On the other hand, there is a much more adequate ethical approach, one that we might call the Catholic approach. The fundamental difference between these two is perceived very early in any ethical analysis. There is a fork in the road right at the beginning. If you go one way, you will end up in one of the three approaches we have considered or in something similar. If you go the other way, you will be in basic agreement with Catholic moral thinking.

This fork in the road represents the choice between two fundamental orientations, two different understandings of man's place in the universe, two different ethical worldviews. One worldview sees man in his relation to the universe in a way that leads toward subjectivism, individualism, and pragmatism. The other worldview understands man's place in the universe in a way that leads to a recognition of objective morality and of certain moral obligations. To make our discussion of these two orientations easier, we will label the first, the one that leads toward subjectivism, as the modern worldview. This is not to say that it is a new view, but that it seems to have become increasingly popular in the modern world. the other can be called the classical worldview. This approach is also very much alive today, though perhaps it was more widespread in the past than at present. This is the ethical worldview of the Catholic Church.

Individuals are not always able to articulate their worldviews, or even be fully conscious of them, but it is this kind of orientation that usually underlies ethical thinking and moral positions. I'd like to explain these orientations by comparing them on a number of different points.

In the first place, there is the question of man's place in the universe, the fundamental question from which everything else seems to follow. In the modern worldview, the emphasis is put on the role of man. Man is perceived at the center of the universe of meaning and value, and man's role is to exercise dominion over the world. Whatever meaning there may be apart from man is not as important as the meaning given to things by man. Man's moral obligations are not defined so much in terms of acceptance and respect as in terms of the need to be wise in the exercise of control. According to this worldview, the world is what man will make of it, and the responsibility is to make the world as good a one as possible for humankind. When God is part of this worldview, He is seen as the Creator who placed man in the world to make it serve him. Man's responsibility to God is fulfilled by using the world for man's benefit.

In the classical worldview, man's role is seen differently. Man, both as the race and as the individual, is seen as a very important part of the universe but not as its center. The world has meaning and value apart from the meaning and value given to it by man. Man's own life has a meaning and purpose, and his moral obligation is to accept, respect, and live in accordance with that meaning and purpose. The will of God is largely expressed in the natural ordering of things. Man fulfills his responsibility to God by respecting nature, especially his own nature, for creation is good and man is sacred.

The importance of this initial difference can be seen in a question such as that of laboratory fertilization of human ova. Someone who adheres to the modern worldview is likely to see no inherent reason to object to this type of procedure. After all, man should continually seek ways of improving his life. On the other hand, a proponent of the classical worldview will be immediately suspicious. To artificially intervene in what is naturally an intimate human process seems to be disrespectful of man's basic goodness.

The weakness of the modern worldview is that it encourages the abuse of man by man, emphasizing as it does man's right to control. The strength of the classical worldview is that it limits man's abuse of man by emphasizing the obligation to respect the inherent goodness in man. It is sometimes mistakenly thought that the modern worldview has a more positive view of man, recognizing his control over creation. It seems to me, however, that the classical worldview puts much more emphasis on the goodness of man, placing him beyond the limits of what we can legitimately manipulate. Man is so good that he cannot be violated, even for the best of motives.

Let us continue to consider some of the differences between the two worldviews. In the context of the modern worldview, the nature of man and the universe does not impose any specific moral obligations. Moral obligations do not come from outside the person; rather, what is right or wrong is *decided* by the individual. There is no such thing as objectively right or wrong actions. Actions, like other things, derive their meaning and value from persons, so the individual must decide for himself which action is better.

In the classical worldview, the individual's obligation is to *discover*, not decide, what is the right thing to do. The universe has a purpose, and that given purpose imposes obligations. There is a certain harmony in the universe. The individual cannot simply decide for himself what is right but must act in such a way that he, too, is in harmony with God's creative will.

The difficulty with the modern worldview is that it is extremely arrogant. To say that actions have no moral meaning until given that moral meaning by man is presumptuous, to say the least. Things do have meaning apart from man; actions do have consequences apart from the meaning given to the actions by man. Man doesn't decide what a particular action will mean in its entirety. He may affect its meaning, but it is not meaningless without him.

The third difference is closely related to what we have just been considering. One of the most fundamental ethical questions is whether the end justifies the means. The end is the purpose, what one hopes to accomplish. The means is the action taken to achieve that purpose. Is a good purpose sufficient reason to act with any type of behavior? The two worldviews give different answers to this question.

As was noted earlier, in the modern worldview the meaning of something is the meaning it has for someone. An action is good or evil depending upon the meaning it has for the one performing the action. And the thing that gives an action meaning is primarily the purpose for which it is being done. A man-centered ethical worldview must focus largely on the purpose or end.

The classical approach, on the other hand, considers actions very important, even apart from the purpose for which they are undertaken. Actions have consequences of their own — consequences which are not always what the person intended and which can be very destructive of human good despite the good purposes they intend to achieve.

The argument for abortion often is made in terms of good purposes. For example, a woman may not want to interrupt a career that she finds rewarding. Certainly, in most circumstances, that constitutes a good purpose. Just as certainly, however, that purpose does not justify killing. The problem with the end-justifies-the-means approach is that it imposes no limits in terms of *what* may be done, because the only way to set limits is to recognize the consequences inherent in actions. Abortion kills whether the purpose is good or evil, and killing destroys respect for human life whether the purpose is good or evil. True moral responsibility involves focusing on actions as well as purposes.

Another difference between the two worldviews is in the language they use in describing the moral situation of the individual. The modern worldview stresses the freedom of the individual. He or she has the right to decide for himself or herself what is the right thing to do; he or she is not bound by objective moral laws; it would be wrong for someone else to impose a moral position on him or her. This emphasis on freedom and rights follows from the denial of objective morality. If there is no objective morality, then we must recognize the freedom of the individual to decide for himself what is right and good.

Those who adopt the classical worldview tend to stress the obligations of the individual rather than his freedom or his rights. The focus is not on the individual, but on the larger context to which he must respond. Since there is an objective morality, an individual cannot make something good which is in itself evil.

It is, of course, important to insist upon individual freedom and individual rights. But, I maintain that too much emphasis on freedom and rights is not conducive to responsible morality. In our culture, we have too often seen this emphasis on "rights" lead to a sort of selfishness, to a concern for what I or my group wants that goes so far as to ignore or deny the needs of others. I sincerely doubt whether real moral responsibility can be taught to children by stressing freedom and rights. This approach is part of a mistaken worldview and fosters moral irresponsibility.

Let us consider the final distinction between the two worldviews. An individual who adheres to the modern worldview, when beginning his moral analysis, tends to consult his own experience and perception. What would this action mean for me, in this situation?

Thus, the whole emphasis is on a particular situation and on what that situation means to the individuals involved. On the other hand, a proponent of the classical worldview begins his moral analysis with rational reflection. What would the contemplated action involve, and what are its implications? Does it conform to the obligation to respect the goodness and order of creation? Individual situations and individual differences are not stressed. Rather, what is necessary is to understand what an action of this kind involves. By withdrawing slightly from the situation and reflecting upon the larger context, it is possible to arrive at guidelines which help to indicate moral obligations.

Once again, the classical orientation seems to have more validity. To begin the decision-making process by dwelling on the circumstances of an individual case is to court the possibility of deciding what is of immediate benefit to the individual rather than of respecting that which will enhance the good for all.

It is not possible to *prove* that one worldview is more valid than the other. It is not a question of proof. Nor can the whole choice between the two be reduced to the fundamental religious question of whether one accepts God or not. While both positions can be religious, they operate according to a very different understanding of man's place in the universe, not to mention his relationship to God.

Though we cannot prove that the classical worldview is more valid, there are compelling reasons for choosing it over the modern worldview. Some of these have already been indicated in the previous discussion. For one thing, the Catholic understanding of God, man, and creation is in much closer agreement with the classical worldview, and it seems foolish to dismiss an understanding that has received such strong support over the ages.

Another important reason for choosing the classical approach over the modern is in terms of the results. The overall validity of an ethical approach can partially be determined by an honest evaluation of the long-term consequences of living according to that approach.

One of the things that the twentieth century will probably be known for is that it has been a century of global wars and totalitarian dictatorships. Few individuals in previous history have had such a destructive impact upon such large numbers of people as have men like Hitler and Stalin. The Nazis in Germany and the Bolsheviks in the Soviet Union both adopted a type of philosophy that more closely resembles the modern worldview than the classical. They held that there are no inherent limits to what is morally acceptable. They, themselves, determined what was right or wrong, and they made those decisions on the basis of what they wanted to achieve. Anything was acceptable as long as it served the desired end. It takes only a little knowledge of history to know the kind of atrocities that this kind of thinking justified.

Many people who base their ethical decisions on the modern worldview are dedicated to the ideal of not hurting others and deeply resent any suggestion that their approach is not very different from the approach of a Hitler or a Stalin. I sympathize with their resentment; they certainly are not Hitlers or Stalins. Yet, in a real way, their approach to moral questions does make it easier for a Hitler or Stalin to work his inequity. If there are no inherent limits to what is acceptable behavior, then it is difficult to say that Hitler went too far. Most of those who advocate a modern worldview do so in defense of freedom and individual fulfillment. But how can an individual claim moral freedom to do his own thing and still maintain a basis from which to tell a Hitler that he cannot do his own thing? As one Protestant ethicist has put it, "Utter freedom in the private sphere can be purchased only at the cost of allowing other men license in the public sphere."[5]

Not everyone who adopts the modern worldview ends up with the same emphasis. We have already seen three different styles — morality as practicality, as opinion, and subjectivity. Each is a type of the modern worldview. A second, more critical look at each of these might provide additional reasons for choosing the *classical* worldview.

Morality as practicality is an example of the end-justifies-the-means approach. What counts is results. The problem is that as soon as we begin to take such a pragmatic approach, we begin to view as important only those results that are tangible or material. Although I can certainly agree that consequences are important, yet emphasizing merely the practical results may not always achieve the most desirable consequences. The practical emphasis will choose consequences in terms of the so-called "standard of living;" it fails to go beyond the tangible and measurable to recognize the importance of values and attitudes. For example, think of what would happen to our moral sensitivity if we did as Hardin suggests — allow much of the world to starve because it is not practical to try to feed them.

If we are really concerned about consequences, we will be concerned with the means used as well as with the desired end. Concentration on the end to be achieved can blind a person to the reality of what he or she is doing. If a woman is considering an abortion to solve the problem of an unwanted pregnancy and if the only consideration that has moral validity is a good purpose or end, then she has no need of further consideration once she has satisfied herself that the abortion would be performed for a good purpose — to prevent difficulties for the child or to make it more probable that she herself will find fulfillment in life. Although these are good goals, at what cost are they to be achieved? And will they, in fact, be achieved by abortion. Simply having a good purpose does not mean that truly good consequences will be produced. In the first place, the very action of abortion produces an evil consequence — the destruction of innocent human life. Secondly, using abortion as a solution to a problem pregnancy contributes to a dangerous tendency in society — to ignore the needs of the weak and the helpless. These evil consequences follow naturally from abortion itself, even though the immediate purpose of the abortion may be a good one. The end-justifies-the-means is a dangerous principle, one that can very easily be used to justify the violation of any individual's life or dignity.

What about morality as opinion? In considering some of the consequences of this approach and the consequences to society of adopting the tolerance ethic, I am particularly struck by the likelihood that proponents of this will end up denying precisely those values that they claim to be defending — individual freedom and responsibility in moral matters. If we can no longer talk about what is right or wrong but only about who decides what is right or wrong, then we no longer have any basis for criticizing someone else's behavior. If a person thinks that an action is right, who am I to consider it wrong. The person is acting according to his opinion, and that is what morality is all about. To suggest that your behavior is wrong would be an intolerable imposition of my moral views on you.

But what do we do when, as a matter of fact, we do think that someone's behavior is wrong as in some types of criminal behavior? If we follow the tolerance ethic, our moral thinking and rhetoric do not permit us to say that he or she did wrong. Instead, we say that he must be "sick" or that social conditions made him act. Of course, to say this is to say that the person is not free and responsible. Thus, in the pursuit of a morality of individual freedom, the tolerance ethic ends up denying that freedom.

There is yet another way in which the tolerance ethic threatens the very freedom of conscience that it seeks to defend. Insisting that everyone has a right to live according to his own conscience implies an obligation on the part of someone else to see that the individual is permitted to do what he claims a right to do. If, for example, every woman has a moral right to have an abortion if she so wishes, then someone else has the obligation to perform that abortion or assist in performing that abortion. But this obligation threatens the so-called "conscience clause" which protects the nurse and others from reprisals if they refuse, on the basis of conscience, to assist at an abortion. And we can expect that it will continue to be threatened as long as the tolerance ethic is widely supported. To insist that I have a right to do whatever I think is right suggests that you are acting unreasonably if you do not provide me with what I need. The theory, of course, is that I can do what I want as long as no one else

16

is hurt. In practice, the emphasis on the first half of that statement is hardly compatible with serious attention being given to the second half. In the name of the woman's freedom of conscience to have an abortion, the nurse's freedom of conscience is being threatened.

Morality as subjectivity also concentrates on the individual who is deciding rather than on the action that is being taken. One of the most basic problems with this whole approach is that it does not attach enough importance on the social impact of our behavior, on the consequences. Social responsibility always needs to be fostered; our hope of being able to live together peacefully in society depends upon individuals accepting social responsibility. But social responsibility can be fostered only by emphasizing actions and the consequences of actions. It is *not* fostering social responsibility to view morality exclusively in terms of subjective attitudes.

As has been indicated, all three approaches to the modern worldview assume that the individual's own perceptions determine what is right and what is wrong. And that is precisely where they are in error. Morality does not depend primarily upon the individual, his motives, or his goals. Some fundamental goods are violated by certain actions, regardless of the reason why a person performs these actions. Only the classical worldview recognizes that the real meaning of things is not dependent upon how they are perceived. Objective truth in morality does exist. To kill an innocent human person directly is a violation of the goodness of life, and it is therefore evil, even if millions say that they do not see it that way. Although we may not always agree exactly on what our objective moral obligations are, there is no hope of a sound morality without recognizing that there is a moral meaning to the universe that we must attempt to discover and abide by. A denial of objective morality leads to individualism, subjectivism, and utilitarianism, and we have seen some indications of where these approaches lead.

Part III — The Decision-Making Process

When an individual is faced with a very personal moral question in an individual situation, he is not always immediately aware of what should be done. At times, it can seem a long way from one's basic ethical orientation — one's worldview — to the concrete decision about what to do here and now. But an acquaintance with the road that must be traveled and of the signposts along the way may make the trip easier.

The first step is to determine some general ethical principles from our analysis of man's place in the universe. By general ethical principles, I mean some statements of value and meaning on various dimensions of life. For example, one such principle is the sanctity of life principle, which incorporates two closely related statements of ethical belief:

1. That human life is sacred by the very fact of its existence; its value does not depend upon a certain condition or perfection of that life.

2. That, therefore, all human lives are of equal value.

Another general principle might be called the sharing-of-resources principle and can be stated in words something like this: The natural resources of the earth are not the exclusive property of individuals or groups to do with entirely as they wish. All men, present and future, deserve to share in the benefit of these resources.

There are many additional general principles that can be derived from the basic understanding of man's place in the universe. One more example — the human sexuality principle — might be mentioned. This principle states that sexual expression has two inherent purposes, one procreative and the other a communication of the total commitment to each other of a husband and a wife. The two are intimately related in the sense that life comes from love. Principles of this sort have been developed as a result of efforts to understand man's purpose.

It is not always easy to take even this first step — the conclusion that respect for creation and the purposes of creation mean such and such. Fortunately, we need not often engage in this kind of enterprise ourselves. Many of the best thinkers over the ages have addressed themselves to these sorts of questions, and many are still continuing to do that. Ordinarily, we can be secure in our attempt to stay on the right path if we follow the wisdom of the ages, especially as it has been conveyed and interpreted by the Catholic Church.

Of course, even at this level not all questions have been answered; general principles must occasionally be reconsidered. But by and large, such endeavors can be left to the Church and to moralists. I am not, by any means, discouraging your own attempts to wrestle with general principles. I am simply indicating that wiser men than you or I and men operating perhaps more under the influence of the Holy Spirit than you or I have already posted some good directions along our path. We must be careful, of course, that the principles we accept are the right ones, not those formulated by proponents of the modern worldview, who have set up their own signposts. Probably the best course is to adhere to the general moral principles taught by the Church.

The second step is to develop more specific moral guidelines from the general principles. What guidelines for behavior follow from principles such as the sacredness of human life, the sharing of resources, and the procreative and unitive purposes of sexuality? Although these principles, as well as others, have a number of applications, I will limit my examples and not attempt to draw the total picture.

One of the behavioral guidelines of the sanctity-of-life principle would be this: It is wrong to unnecessarily endanger one's life or health. This is not necessarily the primary guideline that follows from the sanctity-of-life principle (the first obligation might be the obligation not to kill an innocent human person directly), but it is an example of a specific guideline developed from the general principle. It clearly goes a long way toward indicating the precise implications of saying that human life is good. My obligation is to preserve my health and protect my life, yet life and health are not the only values. If there is sufficient reason for endangering my health, it may be right to do so. Thus, the guideline gives me direction, but it does not resolve all judgmental questions for me. I still have to determine, in a specific case, what constitutes sufficient or proportionate reason for endangering my health.

An example of a guideline that follows from the sharing-of-resources principle is that it is wrong to use *much more* than one needs when others are not having even their minimal and essential needs met. The concept of private property is a justifiable one, but it cannot be used to deprive others who have a great and real need of what we may have in abundance.

An example of a guideline that follows from the principle that sexual love and procreation are inherently linked, that the unitive and procreative purposes of marriage go together is this: It is wrong to separate love-making from life-giving in such a way that new life begins totally separate from sexual love.

In determining guidelines, as in determining general principles, the individual does not need to depend totally upon his own resources. Moral guidelines of this sort have been developed over the ages, and theologians and bishops continue to develop and teach the best guidelines. In fact, it would be irresponsible for an individual to determine entirely for himself what behavioral guidelines follow from general principles. On the other hand, as an important member of the human community and as a contributor to the proper understanding of the Christian message, the individual must think seriously for himself about the implications of general principles. We must think seriously for ourselves and, at the same time, pay careful attention to the wisdom of the ages and the teachings of the Church.

The third step involves analyzing a particular type of action to determine whether or not it is prohibited by the guidelines. For example, does smoking unnecessarily endanger one's health? Or very heavy smoking? Whether and to what extent smoking endangers one's health can be answered on the basis of medical research data. Whether it is an *unnecessary* risk is harder to determine; it depends more on the individual situation and what might be gained from smoking. The third step, then, is basically an analysis of what the action involves rather than what the moral rules are.

Other examples might be helpful. Do kidney transplants from a live donor unnecessarily endanger the person's health? What constitutes unnecessary risks in a context like this? Is artificial insemination with the use of a donor's semen a dehumanizing separation of love-making and life-giving? Does fertilization of a human ovum in a test tube conflict with the purposes of human sexuality? Does the small amount that the U.S. contributes to assistance for underdeveloped countries (approximately 1/5 of 1% of the Gross National Product) violate our obligation to share some of our wealth with those in desperate need? Is the fact that the U.S., with about 6% of the world's population, uses about 40% of the world's natural resources a violation of our obligation to share?

These are examples of the types of questions that have to be asked and answered in the third step. I am not attempting to answer the questions here, because they are often complex and can only be answered well by a very careful analysis of all the factors involved. On some of these questions there may not be agreement even among those who accept the same general principles and moral guidelines (for example, smoking). On others, the Church is unable to offer clear answers as to the application of the moral guidelines (for example, how much use of resources by rich nations is immoral). On still other questions, analyses have produced fairly well-defined answers. For example, it is usually considered acceptable for a live donor to donate an organ provided that there is likelihood of proportionate benefit and provided the functional integrity of the donor is not impaired or seriously endangered. In many of the most important questions in medical ethics today — such as abortion and euthanasia — the Church has formulated a very careful analysis of what precisely is involved. When such agreement has been reached and is seriously taught, the individual is obligated to know that answer and to attempt to understand the reasoning involved. It would be irresponsible to ignore the analysis done by people who have carefully considered all dimensions of the question and who begin from the same starting point.

On the other hand, when the Church has not provided clear analysis, the individual must attempt to do so on his own, with whatever help he can get. Not all precise moral obligations are clearly taught by the Church. For example, though the Church has not conclusively taught that cigarette smoking is or is not an unnecessary endangering of one's health, it remains a moral question.

The fourth step goes beyond an analysis of the type of action involved and the moral implications of that action to a consideration of all important situational factors. The focus is no longer on the act of organ donation, but on this *particular case* of organ donation. The situation is important, and it often makes some difference. I am, of course, not talking about the extreme form of situation ethics which argues that a thing is right or wrong depending upon the situation. For example, a kidney donation might be considered quite acceptable in general, but what about the case where the donor gives his consent only after an enormous amount of pressure has been exerted? This kind of a situational factor might make a big difference in the morality of a particular case of organ donation.

An individual may also have to keep in mind the concept of the lesser evil in a specific situation. For example, assume that we have concluded that heavy smoking is immoral because of the probable damage to health. But suppose an individual is so dependent upon tobacco that he or she cannot function mentally and emotionally without it. In this situation, we might conclude that it would be the lesser evil to continue to smoke. Moral guidelines sometimes include terms like "disproportionate" or "unnecessary." Whether something is disproportionate or unnecessary may depend upon the situation.

The most important point to keep in mind about the situation, though, is this: One must remain morally clearheaded in the situation and not be sidetracked by purely emotional concerns or irrelevant factors. At times, the particular situation may make us aware of important dimensions of a question that have been ignored earlier. It is important to remain open to such possibilities. But one must also guard against the danger of ignoring the most important dimensions of the question as one becomes personally involved in the situation. For example, I have been involved in discussions of abortion where so much has been said about why the woman didn't avoid conception or who should accept financial responsibility that the basic question of whether or not this is justifiable killing is nearly ignored. In the midst of the situation, the desire to seek an easy solution, the temptation to go along with the suggestions of others, the feeling that we should, above all, be practical, and the tendency to forget earlier, more calm, reflections, are all very strong. The individual is obligated not to become so engrossed in the situation that he or she forgets all of his or her prior moral wisdom and convictions.

The final step involves making a decision on what exactly should be done in the specific situation. Even after all that has gone before, it is not always easy to take this final step. Sometimes, even though the individual may know clearly what the proper decision is, it is still difficult for him to follow through. But great strength can be derived from firm and clear convictions. This is another reason to reflect on moral issues long before being faced with them yourself. It can make the decision-making process considerably easier and much less anxious. A firm decision does not, of course, involve arrogance or close-mindedness. It is possible to be understanding of those who disagree, to listen to them seriously, and yet to remain convinced of the rightness of your decision. In the same way, we can give moral advice with firmness and conviction without imposing that position on those who disagree.

When the decision is particularly difficult and when it is not at all clear what the moral principles and guidelines imply, it may be best to get additional help if there is time and opportunity. Everyone who takes morality seriously should be aware of someone whom they can turn to for consultation in moral matters. Such a person should be educated in moral issues and possessed of good moral common sense. (The consultant does not need to be a priest or moralist; however, my chief moral consultant is my wife.) Although conversation with such a person may not resolve all doubts, it can be of considerable help. Certainly, some comfort and support can be derived from knowing that you did your best to get a clear picture of the moral issues. When the decision is very difficult, that kind of support is important.

The actual decision-making process does not always follow the step-by-step progression that I have outlined nor is it always needed. But this kind of systematic analysis makes us aware of what exactly is involved. Some of the biggest problems in moral thinking today arise from the fact that people see only one dimension of a problem or fail to make sure that they are basing their conclusions on correct assumptions. Careful effort in moral decision-making is not always made.

Obviously, it is not an easy task to improve our society's moral thinking, but I have no doubt that some progress can be made. Such progress demands that we all be willing to do careful moral thinking ourselves and to pay careful attention to the wisdom of the ages and the teachings of the Church. We have to be willing to give advice to others and to take public stands. And we have to be willing to understand our contemporary culture and its values.

There is reason for hope. People are not inherently evil or immoral. I would like to quote a passage that encourages me from time to time and which you might want to consider. In writing about the Natural Law (which is another name for the classical approach), J. H. Jacques said:

> "The theory of Natural Law . . . makes us see that morality is in a very real sense natural and normal. Because we generally become aware of moral problems only when we are under the strain of uncertainty and temptation, it is all too easy for us to get the impression that morality is always a matter of

strain and difficulty, and that there is something in goodness which makes it alien to human nature and almost impossible to achieve, whereas most of the time we are carrying out our social and individual obligations without any awareness of the possibility of doing anything else. The theory of Natural Law makes us see that virtues and goodness are normal and sane, and immorality and vice corruptions and perversions of our true nature.

"This is far from saying that everybody is nearly as good as they should be, and that there is nothing seriously amiss with men as individuals and in various social groups. There have been monsters of iniquity, and nations and people possessed of what appears almost as a fever of immorality. Yet, the extraordinary thing is that such monsters have so often wanted their vices to be regarded as virtues, and nations which have followed paths of the most wicked aggression and exploitation have deluded themselves that they were advancing the cause of civilization, fulfilling their destiny, or forwarding the will of God. We are so under the spell of morality that the vilest deeds have to be given a moral justification by those who perpetrate them, and the blackest character tries to convince others that he is an angel of light. This is not just crude hypocrisy. Right conduct has a claim upon us which it is not easy to ignore, and is seldom unaccompanied by at least a vague uneasiness. Goodness is normal."[6]

If people have a proper understanding of what it means to be good, they may not always be good. But often they will be. The biggest task is to improve the quality of ethical thinking in our culture so that vices will not be regarded as virtues.

FOOTNOTES

1. Joseph Fletcher, *The Ethics of Genetic Control: Ending Reproductive Roulette*, Doubleday, NY, NY, 1974, p. 57.

2. Garrett Hardin, "Living on a Lifeboat," *Bioscience*, Vol. 24, October, 1974, p. 561.

3. *Ibid.*, p. 565.

4. Paul Ramsey, *The Patient as Person: Exploration in Medical Ethics*, Yale University Press, New Haven, Conn., 1970, pp. 188-190.

5. Ralph B. Potter, *War and Moral Discourse*, John Knox Press, Richmond, Va., 1969, p. 35.

6. J. H. Jacques, *The Right and the Wrong*, The Society for the Promotion of Christian Knowledge, London, 1965, pp. 90-91.

Ordinary and Extraordinary Means of Prolonging Life

ANTHONY R. KOSNIK, STD

The concept of "ordinary and extraordinary means" is a rather old one in the history of moral thought and development. It dates back to the time of St. Alphonsus, who in the 18th century argued that a man need not submit to the excruciating pain involved in an amputation, even if not submitting was done at the risk of his life. The reasoning behind St. Alphonsus' position was that, in the days prior to anesthesia, no man was or should be expected to submit to that kind of pain or torture.

Through the years, the concept of extraordinary means began to be developed more and more, and different applications of the concept were formualted. In more recent times, Father Gerald Kelly[1] (the most prominent medical moralist in the country during the 1940s and 50s) applied the concept of extraordinary means even to situations in which the disease was not terminal. For example, if a patient was counseled to move to a different climate, such a move could be considered extraordinary means and the patient was morally free to accept or reject the advice.

In 1957, Pope Pius XII made a statement about the kind of care we are obligated to give to our health. He maintained that natural reasoning and Christian morals obligate a man to take the necessary means for preserving his life and health. This duty he has toward himself, God, the human community, and, in most cases, specific persons (obviously, immediate family members) derives from a well-ordered charity, from submission to the Creator, from social justice, and from devotion to the family. In fulfilling this duty, the individual is obliged to use all ordinary means, understood in terms relative to the circumstances of persons, places, times, and culture. In other words by ordinary means he refers to means that do not involve any excessive great burdens for oneself or others. Conversely, any means that would impose a "grave burden" upon oneself or another would render a medication or procedure extraordinary and, thus, not obligatory.

At the same time, a person is not forbidden to take more than strictly necessary steps to preserve life and health, as long as in so doing he does not fail in a more serious duty. Thus, if he so chooses, an individual can elect to use these extraordinary means that do impose a serious burden or difficulty, but there is no strict obligation to do so.

As we read the literature on ordinary and extraordinary means, it is important to attempt to understand the different perspectives that various writers use in approaching this question, as well as the different definitions that they attach to the terms "ordinary" and "extraordinary."

In popular or general literature, the understanding of these two terms, for instance, is predicated on the basis of whether the procedure is simple, easily available, and economically feasible. Thus, a blood transfusion would normally be regarded as an ordinary means. However, if it was a very rare blood type that was difficult to get, this procedure might easily be regarded as an extraordinary means.

In medical literature, the distinction between ordinary and extraordinary is made in terms of what is standard, accepted medical practice in a given community or region. Thus, the question does not depend on how complex or how difficult the procedure is, but on what is the accepted medical practice for that area. For example, highly complex medical centers located in urban areas would apply different standards than would less sophisticated medical facilities located in remote regions. Thus, in the medical literature, "ordinary" procedures refer to standard, accepted medical practice, and "extraordinary" means experimental or exceptionally difficult procedures. For example, psychosurgery — an experimental procedure for controlling violent behavior patterns — is considered an extraordinary procedure. However, as psychotherapy techniques become more sophisticated in the future, what is considered highly experimental now could become standard medical practice. On the other hand, procedures that are considered ordinary in most circumstances (such as the heart transplant) might be considered extraordinary in the case of an elderly patient or a patient with severe complications.

The theological literature defines the terms "ordinary" and "extraordinary" in still another way. Father Kelly, whose definitions of these terms are rather classic, defines ordinary procedures as all medicines, treatments, and procedures which offer a reasonable hope of benefit for the patient and which can be obtained and used without excessive pain or other inconvenience. The criteria he uses to distinguish between ordinary and extraordinary is the proportionality between the hardship that is involved and the hope that it offers to the patient.

Obviously, what constitutes hardship is determined not merely according to medical considerations but also moral, emotional, psychological, social, and family considerations. In 1956, in his *Moral Guidance*,[2] Father Edwin Healy suggested that a procedure that would cost over $2,000 or a procedure that would confine a person for six months to bed or permanently confine him there (i.e., an iron lung or dialysis machine) would constitute an extraordinary hardship and would therefore be considered extraordinary means. Likewise, any procedure that constituted a 10% risk in terms of mortality would be considered a sufficiently grave risk to be regarded as extraordinary. Complications like old age or a weak heart would also serve to render otherwise ordinary procedures extraordinary. Thus, in the 1950s "ordinary" and "extraordinary" means were determined by analyzing the expense involved, the pain or hardship that would result, and the availability or unavailability of the procedures.

The developments of the last decade have almost obliterated the consideration of hardship from this question. For instance, the availability of health insurance and the fact that the community in many instances absorbs the expense eliminates to a great extent the consideration of financial burden. Likewise, modern drugs, surgery, and other procedures can eliminate, to a large extent, the pain consideration. In the same way, the development of medical centers and improved methods of transportation make the availability of even sophisticated procedures readily accessible.

As a result of these developments, the basis for determining extraordinary and ordinary means has shifted from a consideration of the difficulty or the hardship (Pius XII's focus) to a consideration of the hope that a given procedure offers the patient. In other words, the emphasis is now on the person rather than the procedure. So significant has been this shift in emphasis, in fact, that some moral theologians are suggesting that perhaps the time has come to abandon the distinction between ordinary and extraordinary. They reason that so long as mention is made of ordinary and extraordinary means, the focus today should be on the person and thus the primary approach to the question should be made in terms of quality of life judgments.

Father Richard McCormick[3] identifies two situations so affecting the quality of life that they could render any means to prolong that life extraordinary. The first is a continuing condition of minimal or almost nonexistent ability to experience life or relate. The second is the existence of excruciating or intractable pain. Even though pain is one way of experiencing life, excruciating pain so focuses one in upon oneself and drugs so isolate one from others and from the world of experience that if the intractable pain cannot be alleviated, any means for prolonging such a life would no longer be ordinary but extraordinary. Thus, an extraordinary means would be one which provides no hope of resulting in the patient's even minimum ability to experience life relationally or of relieving the excruciating or intractable pain which totally isolates the individual from meaningful life experiences.

Father McCormick, being a very cautious theologian, warns that this emphasis on quality of life should not lead to the conclusion that we are evaluating life itself as though one life is more valuable than another because a certain procedure can imbue it with quality of life. His insistence is that every life is ultimately precious — a gift from God. Determining quality of life does not involve evaluating a life in terms of its mission and the fulfillment of that mission. Secondly, he points that in many cases, even though modern medical technology is very sophisticated, there still exists a substantial degree of doubt. Consequently, where there is real doubt, our overriding and governing concern must be a predisposition in favor of life. In other words, in a doubtful situation, the presumption in favor of life must override all other considerations. Finally, he recognizes the fact that because we are human we will make mistakes. When this happens, rather than reject the principle, we should recognize our mistakes with humility and demonstrate a willingness to learn from them.

I would like to develop more fully what Father McCormick is getting at when he says that for a means to be regarded as obligatory it must offer hope to contribute to the patient's ability to experience life or relational activity at least in a minimal way. I think the real issue is the meaning of human life, the kind of importance we, as Christians, attach to the significance of life. To this end, I would like to share some further general considerations about our vision of human life.

We begin by asserting that God is the Author of human life. He alone has absolute dominion over it. Because He is the Source of life, human life must be considered an ultimately precious gift of God. The fact that life has this distinction of being God's gift endows it with its special dignity and demands of all of us a great reverence for human life.

An interesting experience of a few years ago illustrated to me the manner in which contemporary thinking challenges this idea of the dignity of life. About ten years ago, a group of doctors and scientists were developing a procedure known as amniocentesis to help detect fetal abnormality. Their work had progressed to a point where, in close to 98% of the cases, they could identify a defective fetus and indicate with considerable precision the degree of seriousness of the defect with some 46 different genetic problems. They asked a group of ministers and moralists to help them determine guidelines to be used in counseling people about when to terminate the life of the fetus. In other words, how serious would a defect have to be in order to reach a decision to terminate that life? Putting the question in this way implies that decisions on human life are to be made — in pragmatic terms — of what potential, what promise, what degree of development a particular fetus may offer. If this kind of thinking is followed to its logical conclusion, it could result in a situation where only the most perfect could eventually qualify for the right to life. Such a conclusion substitutes the authority and power of God, the Author of Life, for human standards of pragmatism and the need to meet social expectations.

This experience emphasized for me the need for a deeper appreciation of the fact that God is the author of life. For this reason, all human life must be reverenced and not considered as something in the realm of our ability to manipulate according to our own interests. We are not the masters of life, and we cannot decide to do with our own or others lives exactly as we please. There is more to life than simply what I make of it; what commands our ultimate respect for the dignity of life is the fact that God is its source.

Some of the secular literature in this area implies that such a view of life reflects a particular religious ethic that is representative of moral cowardice, of people who are afraid to make crucial decisions about life. Such a conclusion is possible only to those who have forgotten the corollary to this first truth that God is the Author of Life. The corollary asserts that we are *stewards* of the gift of life, and, as such, have been given the responsibility to care for that life. Consequently, whether we like it or not, we must try to be responsible interpreters of the Will of God with regard to the meaning of life.

Responsible stewardship does not mean that we are afraid to make life/death decisions. It implies, rather, that we know the meaning of life and accept the responsibility to protect and support that meaning. Historically, the Church has viewed this responsibility by asserting that physical life, though worthy of great dignity and respect, is still not the greatest absolute. Let me briefly trace the history of the Church's position on this principle.

For centuries, the Church has supported the idea of a "just" war, and has sent its members off with the reminder that their obligation is to shoot to kill. This has been done out of respect for life — life understood not simply in the sense of an individual human life, but of the kind of conditions that are necessary to maintain the quality of life for a large segment of society. Likewise, the Church for centuries has condoned capital punishment as the only effective way of protecting the life of the community. In other words, the Church has upheld the right of society to eliminate one who is a threat to the life of others. Legitimate self-defense has also been regarded as adequate justification for terminating the life of another. Thus, we see that physical life has never been regarded by the Church as the greatest value.

We have to search for a deeper meaning, a deeper purpose, to guide us in making decisions in regard to life. We find this deeper meaning in the words of Christ when He says that we must "love the Lord, your God, with your whole heart and mind and soul and love your neighbor as yourself." This kind of love is the "greatest good" which Pius XII talked about when he said that if we concentrate all our efforts simply on maintaining physical life, we can lose sight of the more fundamental purpose of life — the ability to experience or give expression to that commandment of love which requires consciousness and relationality. Thus, the ability to love becomes the critical value which gives life its meaning and ultimate purpose.

In applying this principle to decisions about ordinary and extraordinary means, it means that we must bring to that decision a Christian vision of what it means to be human. First of all, because life is more than physical existence, it is necessary to consider also the emotional, phychological, and spiritual well-being of the individual. Secondly, we are not obliged to make extraordinary sacrifices in order to preserve mere physical existence. In this respect, Father McCormick says that "if the potential for human relationship is nonexistent, or would be utterly submerged and undeveloped in the mere struggle to survive,"[4] then we can say that that person's God-given life mission has been accomplished. The question is not whether this life is of less value than another; it has its source in God and is ultimately precious. But in attempting to interpret the will of God in regard to life, we must base our interpretation on His own commandment, which is love. If there is no capacity for that, then it is reasonable to conclude that the God-given mission for that life has been accomplished.

We can see how this principle would apply in the case of an acephalic infant, which is developing without a brain and with no capacity for consciousness or relationality. The implications of such a condition, in terms of any surgery that might be needed to continue the person's existence, would be pretty clear. Such means would obviously be regarded as extraordinary and nonobligatory. Special caution needs to be exercised when applying these criteria to other infants. First, in dealing with an infant or fetus, we have no clear indication of what their life mission or value is. Since they are incapable of giving any indication about their mission in life, either from their past life or from the testimony of relatives, every decision represents risky judgment in terms of what is God's will. The second reason for extreme caution is the unpredictability of recovery and the aura of mystery that surrounds life at the very beginning. Certainly, more caution must be exercised in dealing with an infant than when dealing with a patient who has lived a rather full life and has had many opportunities to achieve his mission in life. Generally speaking, there is less possibility of error in judgment in the case of a comatose, terminal 70-year-old than there is at the very beginning of life.

The above remarks make it clear that in contemporary medical practice, the distinction into "ordinary" versus "extraordinary" means cannot be reduced to a neat list of medications or procedures that will always be regarded as "ordinary" or "extraordinary." At times, the simple use of oxygen may be an extraordinary means as in the case of an irreversibly comatose and terminal patient. In another situation, the use of the respirator and other highly complicated and specialized procedures may be judged to be ordinary means if they provide genuine hope of sustaining or supporting conscious relational life. The soundest basis for a good moral decision remains a deep appreciation of the Christian meaning of life and a recognition of the obligation to make every decision a serious attempt to interpret God's will and to respond to the divine plan for that life. Christians dare not approach such a momentous decision without consultation, reflection and prayer.

FOOTNOTES:

1. Gerald Kelly, *Medico-Moral Problems*, Part 5, The Catholic Hospital Association, St. Louis, MO, 1954, p. 8.

2. Edwin Healy, SJ, *Moral Guidance*, Loyola, Chicago, IL, 1943, pp. 162-163.

3. Richard McCormick, "To Save or Let Die," *America*, July 13, 1974, pp. 6-10.

4. *Ibid.*

Ethical Decision-Making

SISTER FRANCESCA LUMPP, CSJ

My specialization field in nursing is nursing service administration. Therefore, I will talk about ethical decision-making from a management point of view.

How competent are professional nurses as decision-makers? When many of us were being educated as nurses, we were being trained to be procedure-followers rather than decision-makers. The decisions we made were based largely on rules and procedures rather than on our own initiative or ingenuity. Consequently, as professional nurses, we did not have much experience in making decisions.

Nursing education has come a long way in the past decade, and, now, many nurse theorists distinguish the uniqueness of the nurse by her ability to make nursing judgments. Nursing education programs are now educating nurses in this area of judgment or decision-making. Therefore, let us reflect on how we make decisions.

In his book, *Management: Tasks, Responsibilities, Practices*, Peter Drucker says, "A decision is a judgment. It is a choice between alternatives."[1] When we make a decision, therefore, we choose a certain course of action based on a particular set of alternatives.

There are four steps to follow in the decision-making process. From the definition given above, it is apparent that the first step is to identify the alternatives. The second step is to evaluate the alternatives, weighing the value of each. Third, we must choose one alternative and, in so doing, make the decision. Lastly, we must convert the decision into action. Let us examine each of these steps in greater detail.

In identifying the alternatives, it is important to remember that there are probably many alternatives for each decision that is made. In this respect, Koontz and O'Donnell in their book *Principles of Management*, say: "If there seems to be only one way of doing a thing, that way is probably wrong."[2] Rarely, are a number of alternatives lacking.

Alternatives begin as ideas, opinions, and sometimes as facts. The person who is responsible for presenting a particular alternative to the group is also responsible for substantiating its relevance. Since alternatives spring from many different sources, they may not always be in agreement. The wise decision-maker must be able to reflect

31

upon all the alternatives, even those in apparent conflict. Peter Drucker warns against "the trap of being right."[3] If the manager thinks that one alternative is right before he or she has even started to view all of the alternatives, probably a good decision will not be made. Thus, the element of conflict or of disagreement is a very important one, in terms of decision-making.

A good manager is one who can tolerate differences; who is not surrounded by people who think the same way as he/she does. It is very beneficial for a management team to be able to openly disagree, for it is in reconciliation of conflicting viewpoints that the most tenable decisions are often made.

After identifying all relevant alternatives, the next step is to evaluate each. This entails thoroughly examining and weighing the value of each alternative that has been identified. Some alternatives will be eliminated because of the "limiting factor."[4] In nursing, the limiting factor frequently is human resources. Thus, it is necessary to realistically evaluate factors that limit certain alternatives and to eliminate these choices because of their impracticality.

Another factor that should be operative in evaluating alternatives is striving for the "optimal" in selecting an alternative. The optimal decision is usually difficult to achieve. Management authors talk about what they term a "satisficing decision;"[5] a decision in which we choose the alternative that will cause the least waves, that will be good enough to get us by, but will really not be the best. The optimal decision requires courage and is hard to execute. However, in choosing, the brave decision-maker strives for the optimal, even though it may be difficult to implement.

The third step in the decision-making process is selecting the appropriate alternative. Management experts caution us to make a "rational" decision, in other words, a decision which will lead most directly to the goal we're trying to achieve. For example, let us say that our goal in a nursing department is to render the most scientifically correct and individualized nursing care possible. Further, in terms of individualized care, our goal is to emphasize the patient's psycho-spiritual needs and to implement the kind of program that will help the patient achieve the degree of wellness that's possible for him or, if not, a degree of acceptance of the illness. If this is the goal, the "rational" decisions made will be those that further the achievement of that goal. Often, however, decisions are made not because they further the achievement of that goal, but rather for the convenience of physicians or for the convenience of the institution.

After selecting an alternative, the fourth and final step is implementing the decision. If as many people as possible have been involved in the first three steps — identifying, evaluating, and selecting the alternatives — many of the problems that might arise in the implementation stage will be eliminated, because people will be aware that a change is going to be made.

Drucker points out three questions that must be asked before implementing the decision: 1) Who has to know about the decision? 2) What actions have to be taken to carry it out? and 3) Who has to take the actions?[6] In the area of moral decision-making, we should reflect on these questions since often nurses are not involved in the first three moral decision-making steps, but are on the front line when it comes to implementation. When a serious moral decision has been made, it is frequently the nurse who has to know about the decision. The actions that must be taken are often nursing activities, and the person who has to perform these actions is the nurse. For example, in the case of Karen Quinlan, the moral decision was made in the legal arena, and one never read anything about ideals and values of the nurses who were taking care of the patient each day.

Since nurses are frequently the people who have to carry out the decisions that are made, there is a real need for nurses who are specialists in the area of nursing ethics. Together with theologians and physicians, nurses must become active participants on medical-moral committees in hospitals and other institutions. Nursing input is lacking because nurses do not feel secure enough to speak on medical-moral issues. There is a great need for critical care nurses and operating room nurses to become knowledgeable about medical ethics. What can be done to encourage and support active and informed participation on the part of nurses? First of all, nurses must begin to provide input to Program Committees of their professional organizations on district, state, and national levels.

In addressing ethical issues in the professional forum, we must speak for the Judeo-Christian position. There are many ethical workshops where the Christian viewpoint is not addressed. We must be fearless in saying that life is sacred because it is created by God. It is necessary that those whose approach to ethics is purely scientific hear us say that the faith dimension is essential in approaching all ethical issues.

What else can we do to educate ourselves more fully in terms of medical ethics? Sources of helpful literature are The Hastings Report published bimonthly by Hastings Center, Institute of Society, Ethics and The Life Sciences, 360 Broadway, Hastings-on-the-Hudson, New York 10706 and The Kennedy Institute, Georgetown University, 36th and "O" Streets, NW, Washington, D.C. 20007. In addition, the Joseph P. Kennedy, Jr. Foundation is offering fellowships to nurse faculty members to study medical ethics.

Because of the interest shown by nurses attending these institutes, the future looks hopeful. I envision the time rapidly approaching when nurses will take an active part in medical-moral decision-making.

FOOTNOTES:

1. Peter F. Drucker, *Management: Tasks, Responsibilities, Practices,* Harper and Row Publishers, New York, 1973, p. 470.

2. Harold Koontz and Cyril O'Donnell, *Principles of Management, An Analysis of Management Functions,* McGraw-Hill Book Co., New York, 1972, p. 174.

3. Drucker, *op. cit.,* p. 474.

4. O'Donnell, *op. cit.,* p. 175.

5. *Ibid.,* p. 174.

6. Drucker, *op. cit.,* p. 476-477.

Ethical Decision-Making

CARL L. MIDDLETON, JR.

Medical-ethical decision-making is a highly complex process. Often, decisions must be made on the spot, and they must be correct. Just as a driver in the Indianapolis 500 race doesn't simply walk to his car and automatically attain the skill needed to drive in the race, so also nurses excel in their own sphere of activity in direct proportion to the efforts they have expended during their training. Their daily moral decisions are sometimes made as spontaneously as the race car driver's decision; ordinarily, no long deliberate reflection precedes them. Rather, they flow almost automatically from the kind of person the nurse is, from the kind of values she has, and from the kind of conscience she has formed within herself over the years.

In any type of reflection on decision-making, especially medical-moral decision-making, I think it is necessary to reflect on the meaning of conscience. By conscience, I am referring both to the individual conscience and also to what might be called the institutional conscience as it relates to medical-moral decision-making. The Second Vatican Council defines conscience as "the most sacred core and sanctuary of man, where he is alone with God whose voice echoes in his depths. In a wonderful manner, conscience reveals that law which is fulfilled by love of God and neighbor. In fidelity to conscience, Christians are joined with the rest of man in the search for truth and for the genuine solutions to the numerous problems which arise in the life of individuals and from social relationships."[1] What does this quotation from Vatican II really mean? To me, it means that conscience represents God's invitation to us to be co-partners in the continuous drama of creation, sharing His love with the persons involved in our lives. Conscience is our ability to respond as free human beings capable of love. Fundamentally, it is a capacity for working out, in communion with God and others, the future of humankind.

Now, if conscience is our ability to respond as free human beings capable of love, what does it mean to be conscientious? Father Nicholas Lohkamp, in an article "Conscience Equals Response-Ability," says that conscientiousness is not doing merely what we are told to do, but rather inventing ways of pleasing, of returning love, of giving worthy gifts to someone who loves us very much and never ceases to do good things for us.[2] Thus, conscience is response. It represents the ability to respond to God in love and to share God's love with others in everyday life. It does not refer to a Freudian understanding of conscience as a feeling of guilt, worry, dissatisfaction, or restlessness. Rather, it refers to a person's sense of right or wrong and the awareness of his responsibility to enter into relationship with God and his fellow men.

Basically, God is present in conscience in three ways. The first way He is present is in our sense of what ought to be. Deep in us there is a consciousness of how things ought to be which keeps us strangely uncomfortable with things the way they are. In this way, God reveals himself and awakens trust and response in the individual. Such response is what we call a person's faith, and this faith response enables us to participate in the joy of love and the life of Jesus and His Church.

However, the Second Vatican Council warns us that there can be no dichotomy between what we believe or profess to believe and how we live. What we profess to believe must be an integral part of our life — lived and manifested in everything we do, everything we say, and everything we become.

The second important way that God impresses conscience is through the individual's realization that he must do something about the way things are and the way they ought to be. We must try and see the full meaning of each situation and must make a specific decision in a response that is both free and of faith. In every moment and every situation, the individual must grapple with the question of what is the right and loving thing for me to do in relationship to God, His Church, and His community. In terms of our responsibility to respond, the Vatican fathers tell us that we are ultimately responsible for making our own moral decisions. Consequently, since each person makes moral decisions that are compatible with his conscience, there is a legitimate diversity in approaches to moral problems.

The third way in which God is present in conscience is through reflection on the actual act of doing what we realized had to be done in order to bridge the gap between what is and what ought to be. Reflecting on the specific ways in which we have addressed ourselves to particular situations helps us grow deeper in love of God and others.

Therefore, conscience is not a static given, not an established list of do's and don'ts; rather, it is a capacity that must be continuously enriched. A good Christian conscience is not synonomous with pat formulas or exact answers to every moral dilemma or every medical-moral problem. Rather, conscience acknowledges the freedom and responsibility to make creative decisions; it expects and respects a certain amount of ambiguity and legitimate diversity as healthy signs of a generation coming together to search for truth and for the general solution to the numerous problems which arise in the life of individuals. Conscience is our inviolable right, and we must follow our well-formed Christian conscience.

The proper formation of consicience is a lifelong task, but how do we go about it? If as Christians we view conscience as a person's ongoing dialogue with God and humankind, it is apparent that a well-formed Christian conscience is constantly in tune with God in whatever ways He speaks to us. St. Paul informs us that He speaks to us in a variety of ways.

One way is through sacred scripture. The Christian Catholic certainly cannot be indifferent to this source of revelation from God to His people. With St. Jerome, we must recognize that "he who is ignorant of the scriptures is ignorant of Christ." However, we must also recognize that the Bible does not provide a complete ethical code. For example, the Bible is silent on a number of critical moral questions, such as the definition of death, the morality of a heart transplant, thermonuclear war, technological pollution, poverty, energy, etc.

But the Bible does offer an indispensible understanding of the fundamental meaning of morality and conscience. It presents the role of conscience in a way that no pagan philosopher or modern psychologist has ever dared conceive it. It sees the role of conscience not as conformity to abstract inflexible law but as the individual human response to an invitation from a personal, loving God. Certain basic moral truths recur again and again in scriptures, such as God's loving concern for man, especially the poor and the sick; the special reverence for life and for human beings, particularly for the sinner and the outcast; the significance of suffering and death that can transform these tragedies into creative experiences.

Such scriptural themes demand repeated reflection and help us assume the conscience of Him who is our ultimate norm: Jesus Christ. Because Jesus Christ is the ultimate norm of morality, we are called to be a people of love just as Jesus was a person of love. Jesus' love was unique in that it did not expect to be loved in return. In other words, He totally gave of himself to others without asking them to give Him something in return, and we are called to love in the same way.

In speaking about the importance of continued reflection on scripture, Richard McCormick says if the light of the Gospel can aid in the discovery of truly human solutions to our problems, then those who have the Gospel have a source of knowledge which others not exposed to the Gospel do not have. Whatever material content this light of the Gospel leads to it will always be utterly human, not beyond or at variance with the human and the reasonable.[3] In other words, the more we grow in the values and attitudes of the Gospel, the more fully human we become, because the Gospel talks about basic human values. Therefore, as Christians, we are called to put on Jesus Christ the Lord, who is the ultimate in normal reality. This can be done only through continual and ongoing reflection and meditation on the values and energies that Jesus came to share with us.

The second way in which God speaks to us and thus an important source of conscience formation is the Church's magisterium. Through the centuries, the Church has proven itself the most effective and consistently reliable teacher of moral truth known to man. In today's complex and confused world, there is greater need than ever for the Church to provide authoritative guidance and direction for her people. The promised assistance of the Holy Spirit, the Church's long experience and universal presence, and her accessibility to the best minds available make her ideally suited for this task.

As we have seen earlier however, this does not mean that the Church can provide us with all the answers. Rather, it means that we should be attentive to the Church's teachings and make an effort to determine precisely what the magisterium of the Church is currently saying on a given issue. Thus, we should strive not only to obey the Church's law but to examine the values that the law presents and appropriate them for our lives.

In addition, as Catholic Christians we must acknowledge that the presumption of truth is with the Church's teaching office, and we must approach her teachings with this presumption in mind. In other words, we can't do our "own thing" and say, "Oh, what do they know?" We must be open, and we must study, and we must know exactly and precisely what the Church is teaching.

It is important, however, to recognize the limitations of the Church's magisterial teaching and, when formulated Church teaching is inadequate or incomplete, to exercise our right and responsibility to bring this fact to the attention of the magisterium. The American bishops have spelled out this responsibility in their pastoral letter, *Human Life in Our Day*, in which they issued norms for legitimate theological dissent. They stated: "The expression of theological dissent from the magisterium is in order only if the reasons are serious and well-founded, if the manner of the dissent does not question or impugn the teaching authority of the Church, and is such as not to give scandal."[4] In other words, openness to the magisterium in the formation of one's conscience does not mean putting on a straightjacket and abandoning one's own moral responsibility. Rather, we must make a serious commitment to grow with the Church in struggling to resolve the problems of all mankind. Precisely for this reason we need to be attentive to the variety of ways the Church's teaching manifests itself.

38

What are some of these ways? First and foremost, the Church promulgates her teaching through ecumenical councils, such as the Second Vatican Council. Other sources of teaching include the Papal Encyclicals, allocutions, statements and addresses by the Holy Father, such as *Humanae Vitae*. Next would be documents, statements, and responses from Roman congregations, such as the recent Vatican statement on sexuality. Then, there are the statements of a particular country's bishops such as the U.S. Catholic Conference of Bishops' document, *Ethical and Religious Directives for Catholic Health Facilities*. U.S. Catholics also have diocesan directors' statements and advisories from the local bishop, such as the local bishop's pastoral letters.

The medical community also has its teaching office or teaching authority. Consequently, in forming our conscience we must be aware of the "magisterium" of the medical community. We must know the medical community's official stand in regard to medical-moral values. Some of the sources of the medical community's moral code include the oath of Hippocrates, the pledge of Florence Nightingale, the statement of the American Colleges of Surgeons on certain unethical practices in surgery, the declaration of Geneva, the declaration of Helsinki, the International Code in Medical Ethics, etc. Thus, we must inform ourselves not only about the Church's teachings but also about the official medical-moral stand of the medical and nursing communities.

The third major way of forming our conscience is through science. Some scientists, better known as "humanists," would like to enthrone reason and science as the only reliable source of ethical decision-making. However, scientific truth represents only a partial understanding of what makes for a fully formed Christian conscience.

Undoubtedly, God's book of nature and creation — science's laboratory — is a vast and limitless treasury of unexplored and undiscovered truth through which God continues to speak to man. To ignore the findings of science would be to ignore the creation of God. No reliable ethical decision can be made without taking into account the evidence that modern science can provide.

However, to think that reason and science have an exclusive monopoly on God's truth and that they alone exhaust the mystery that is man is absurd. Although science has developed great benefits for mankind, it has also made possible the horrors of modern warfare, technological pollution, scarcity of energy, easy abortion, economic inequality, and other moral dilemmas. Thus, to presume that what can be done technologically ought to be done is to forget an important historical lesson and perhaps to prepare the way for man's demise.

In order to make sound moral decisions, we must attempt to see the whole picture, the totality. Science is part of this picture and therefore it is essential to consult the evidence of modern science in order to properly inform our conscience. There are a variety of resource centers that attempt to bring together significant scientific facts and reflect upon them theologically. In addition, certain journals also attempt to present the important salient facts of science and theology and the way in which these facts affect medical-moral issues. We must continually research all input for its validity if we are to arrive at the kind of moral decisions that will help people become the people that they are called to be.

The fourth major source of conscience formation is the Spirit. Christian Catholics are expected to take seriously Christ's promise of the Spirit ("I shall ask the Father and He will give you another Advocate to be with you forever, the Spirit of Truth. . . ." Jn 14:16). If baptism means anything, if the Divine Indwelling is a reality, if Christ's promise that the Spirit will teach us all truth is valid, if St. Paul's insistence that it is by the grace of Christ that we are fashioned in His likeness holds true, then the importance of prayer and sacramental life to the proper formation of conscience becomes clear.

This does not mean that a formed conscience is synonomous with a personal inspiration or revelation from God. Christ speaks to us and we hear Him only after we have opened our hearts to Him. Although scripture, the Church, and modern science cannot be ignored, all the wisdom of the world will never equal the Christian conscience, because it is ultimately God who causes growth. To form our Christian conscience, therefore, we must reflect on the facts and open ourselves to the guidance of authority, but we dare not forget that it is ultimately Christ who forms us. To do this, it is absolutely essential that we pray.

The next important way of forming conscience is through sincerity. Many moderns would like to reduce the meaning of conscience to sincerity. Although there can be no doubt that being true to oneself is the inescapable touchstone of true character and an indispensable foundation for a well-formed conscience, the mark of geniune sincerity is its ability to open up a person to true knowledge and discovery of self.

As people trying to grow deeper in love of God and others, we must strive to find out who we really are and to be the honest, authentic persons we were created to be. One paradox of being human is that we cannot discover who we are by looking exclusively inward. We can be true to ourselves only insofar as we recognize our destiny and reach outward to other persons.

The danger in reducing conscience to sincerity is that conscience formation is thereby turned into personal introspection, with the hope that one will find within himself the answers to the mystery of man. Even if such self-analysis was totally objective, it would still be a very limited and narrow perspective from which to make judgments concerning the welfare of all humankind.

The final important source of conscience formation is community. St. Paul tells us in his epistle to the Phillipians, 1:9, "My prayer is that your love for each other may increase more and more and that it may never stop improving your knowledge and deepening your perception so that you can always recognize what is best." St. Paul's observation about conscience is interesting. We sharpen our conscience, deepen our understanding of what is right, and find out what God expects of us by looking to and loving our neighbor. In other words, a Christian conscience can never be formed apart from the Christian community.

One reason for this is that Christ ordinarily manifests his will not to the individual Christian but through the Christian community. God makes us holy and saves us not as individuals having no mutual bonds, but by making us into a single people. The Second Vatican Council assures us that the Christian community, the people of God, can be an infallible source of God's truth. Even where such universal agreement does not exist, the Christian community provides a reliable testing ground where uncertain and conflicting ideas can be tried, clarified, and refined.

Although the Church's teachers — the theologians and authentic magisterium — can assist the individual Christian in his search for truth by providing accurate insight and practical applications to his life, conscience formation demands more than information. Not only must the mind be instructed, but the person must be transformed. One doesn't become a Christian merely by knowing what is right. The Christian community provides the context in which Christian moral values are experienced and assimilated, and it creates the atmosphere necessary for forming attitudes and convictions. This is why we say that a Catholic hospital is called to be a healing environment, a community of persons who help heal one another through their love and concern for each and every person. Without the example and encouragement that a healing Christian community provides, there is little hope for effective Christian formation of conscience.

Finally, it is necessary to point out that to be Christian is to be community-oriented. The great commandment that summarizes Christianity demands both love of God and of neighbor. Therefore, no one forms a Christian conscience alone; this would be a contradiction. Thus, attempts to interpret individual freedom of conscience as implying absolute autonomy or complete independence from the Christian community misinterpret the whole Christian message. In Galatians 5:13-18, St. Paul says, "My brothers, you were called, as you know, to liberty; but be careful or this liberty will provide an opening for self-indulgence. Serve one another, rather, in works of love, since the whole of the law is summarized in a single command: Love your neighbor as yourself. If you go snapping at each other and tearing each other to pieces, you had better watch or you will destroy the whole community." Without the Christian community, there can be no Christian conscience.

If Christians are by definition lovers, not loners, what changes must we make in our Catholic hospitals in order to have them reflect the love of Christianity? How can we justify breakdowns in communication and the little everyday acts of selfishness that impede our ability to function as a team and deliver effective health care in a truly Christian and healing manner?

We have outlined six major ways of forming consciences. However, the difficulty with ethical decision-making is that we tend to use one of these sources to the exclusion of all the others. For example, a biblical fundamentalist might use the Bible as his sole criteria in decision-making; or, as often happens in the past, some Catholics might rely exclusively on magisterium. To make truly valid ethical decisions, we must use all six of these sources.

To assign medical-moral responsibility to the decisions of the administrator, or chaplain, or doctor, or to think that we can accept the "Directives" as a complete and absolutely certain set of answers for all problems is to reveal a lack of the basic humility and honesty which is demanded of all Christian Catholics. Responsibility for the medical attitudes or conscience formation of a Catholic health facility is shared by the total community. Everyone in the community of a Catholic health care facility is responsible for the moral decision-making and the moral attitudes of that hospital. Therefore each and every person must participate in the process of conscience formation if the institution can be said to be truly moral.

This reality will call for new modes of interaction and new procedures for shared decision-making that will foster ongoing conscience formation. In other words, nurse X cannot just make a decision in isolation from everyone else. Somehow that decision will affect not only the patient but other members of the health care team as well. The point is, do we have a vehicle which will enable us to come together as a community and reflect upon the quality of the medical-moral decisions being made in our institution?

Fidelity to the traditional Catholic concept of respect for the uniqueness of the individual and the freedom of the well-formed conscience may create some difficulties in terms of reconciling this concept with the institution's responsibility to give corporate witness to the constant unchanging values of Christianity. To bridge this gap between personal conscience and institutional conscience, we need an instrument that is flexible enough to respond to the needs of individuals and to the varying situations of hospitals without compromising their basic mission. A Christian Ethical Perspectives Committee might provide such an instrument.

As part of my doctoral work, I have just completed a two-year study on the use of such a committee in Catholic health care facilities. From my experience in forming and working with such a committee, I suggest that this committee should be responsible for establishing and directing an ongoing process of conscience formation that would reflect the following: 1) A concern for the total well-being of every patient. 2) A recognition of the complexity and ambiguity of many health care decisions; it is increasingly difficult today for any one person to make these decisions because the necessary input must come from various sources. 3) A respect for the prevailing pluralism within theology and medicine. 4) Recognition of the community's need to come together to identify and assess key problems in the community and to suggest possible solutions that would provide more effective health care delivery. 5) A continuing appreciation of ongoing developments in medicine and theology. 6) An awareness of the collegial nature of the Church and a corporate sense of responsibility for its mission. 7) A serious effort to integrate respect for personal conscience with fidelity to the institution's mission to witness Christian values. 8) A commitment to moral responsibility as a deeply rooted way of life and not merely as a docile conformity to a static code. To work toward such a renewal should be the primary function of a Christian Ethical Perspectives Committee.

The purpose of a Christian Ethical Perspective Committee would be five-fold. The first and foremost task of the committee would be to assume responsibility for educating the total hospital community concerning medical-moral trends that affect health care. This educational task could be accomplished through lectures, discussions, conferences, workshops, inservice training, and through the use of audio tapes, video tapes, slides, movies, etc. In this area of education and conscience-formation, emphasis on particular decisions would not be as important as the development of a deeper sense of fundamental values.

The second purpose of the committee would be to provide a forum for sharing, exchanging, and coordinating the efforts of all hospital personnel relative to medical-moral values. This forum would encourage staff members to build up mutual trust and cooperation, provide them with an opportunity of bringing up practical problems that pertain to various members of the health care team, and offer them a chance to share and, thus, to alleviate some of the frustrations that are experienced by people working in highly compartmentalized and departmentalized institutions.

A third major purpose would be to provide direction and assure consistency in interpreting and applying policy. However, the committee ought not to become a decision-making body for particular cases. Rather, it should seek constantly to clarify the framework and limits within which decisions can be made. Specific sub-committees could be appointed to facilitate the particular decisions that have to be reached.

Fourth, the committee can act as a channel of communication from the front line of nursing experience to the real line of policy-making. The reason why the "Ethical and Religious Directives" are inadequate is because of a breakdown in communication between those actually involved in the health care delivery system and our bishops. A committee like the one being proposed could re-establish that line of communication by sharing its experiences, problems, and complex decisions, and by making recommendations for improving or modifying the "Ethical and Religious Directives."

The fifth purpose of a Christian Ethical Perspective Committee would be to act as legislative watchdog. As such, the committee must be sensitive to the moral implications of state and federal legislation as it affects the health care apostolate. By becoming sensitive to the moral consequences of legislative developments, the health care facility could use the tremendous power that a hospital community has in terms of its board of trustees and community members to help stave off legislation that would adversely affect the health care apostolate.

To effectively accomplish its mission, the committee's membership should include representatives from every area of health care. A typical committee might include the following representatives: Administration, board of trustees, medicine, obstetrics, gynecology, surgery, psychiatry, neurosurgery, nursing, social services, pastoral care, legal council, and moral theology. Other representatives in the community could also be made members. However, care must be employed when establishing the committee. If ill-begotten, poorly prepared, and inadequately formed, it can become a source of increased tension and conflict in the community. Well-formed, it can be an indispensable means of making the Catholic health facility a living, dynamic sacrament of Christ's healing presence to the world. This kind of committee can provide an environment that helps the community discern basic human values through the sources God uses to speak to us: Scripture, magisterium, science, Spirit, sincerity, and the Christian community.

The Catholic health care facility that forms its conscience in this manner certainly does not view conscience as a lifeless conformity to rules and laws, but rather as a response to the never-ending call to love addressed to us by God. This kind of ongoing process of conscience formation, not only for individuals but as an entire institution, renders us better able to make truly responsible ethical decisions that are responsive to human needs and that fulfill, at the same time, the institution's mission to heal as Jesus did, with love, sincerity, mercy, and forgiveness.

FOOTNOTES:

1. *The Constitution on the Church in the Modern World*, para. 16, The Second Vatican Council.

2. Nicholas Lohkamp, OFM, "Conscience Equals Response-Ability," *Conscience in Today's World*, Jeremy Harrington, OFM ed., St. Anthony Messenger Press, 1970, Cincinnati, Ohio, p. 32.

3. Richard A. McCormick, SJ, "Notes on Moral Theology," *Theological Studies*, Baltimore, Maryland, March 1971, Vol. 32, No. 1, p. 74.

4. *Human Life in Our Day: Pastoral Letter of American Bishops*, ed. by John B. Sherrin, United States Catholic Conference, Washington, D.C., Nov. 15, 1968, p. 18.

Nursing and Pastoral Care

ROBERT D. WHEELOCK, OFM Cap.

Persons involved in pastoral care have a unique opportunity to observe the profession of nursing, and they consider nurses as those persons who truly deliver health care to patients. Physicians order care; nurses give it. Perhaps this is a bit of an over-simplification, and it in no way is meant to play down the importance of the therapists and technicians who are also directly involved in patient care. It is mentioned simply because it points out an important consideration in pastoral-ethical issues; namely, that pastoral people see the nurse as the person with whom they must be most closely allied in their ministry. The public immediately recognizes both nurses and religious health care professionals as people who, by their very profession, claim to be caring and concerned.

Pastoral Assumptions

Several pastoral assumptions should be taken into consideration while reading this article.

First: It is presumed that the reader is a Christian nurse who brings to her work the Christian value system and the power of God's active life of Grace in her person.

Second: It is further assumed that the nurse is dedicated to the nursing profession as a profession of genuine care and concern.

Third: Nurses have a sense of ministry or mission in their work. This refers again to the concept of nursing being more than merely a means of earning money. Perhaps a note on ministry should be interjected here. There are many ways to define ministry, and an individual's concept of the Church certainly affects his definition. However, whichever approach is used, the definition of ministry should include these three points: a) Ministry makes real, concrete, and tangible, the b), special presence of God in the world (an eschatological presence that is not limited by time or space), and c) those who perform this ministry do so in the name of the Christian community. Perhaps in the not too distant future, pastors will commission persons working in health care and other social apostolates to continue to do so in the mane of the Christian community from which they come and to occasionally report to the community the many good things happening in their ministry. In this way, the whole community can be called to a closer involvement in this important work.

Fourth: The nurses's competency in her profession is accepted as a given. To be competent is not synonomous with being cold, hard, and exact. The competent nurse must act in extremely stressful situations and, at times, may have to maintain a certain emotional distance from a particular patient. But there is no reason why a competent nurse, male or female, cannot be a warm and sensitive person. Competency is crucial in a profession that deals with human lives.

Fifth: The fifth assumption is that the nurse is growth-oriented, meaning that she continues to study, read journals, attend meetings, and be actively involved in professional associations. In the scientific fields today, failure to grow is to fall hopelessly behind.

Sixth: Finally, we assume that the nurse finds her profession a fulfilling one. Although there may be times and days when the emotional or physical strain will make it seem otherwise, in general the nurse considers nursing fulfilling.

Areas of Concern

Three major areas of concern that we would like to address ourselves to in this article are: 1) The patient and the families of patients; 2) the nurse; and 3) means whereby the departments of pastoral care and nursing might cooperate more fully in order to achieve better patient care.

The Patient and the Families of Patients

Under this category, we will consider two general areas of concern. First, we will deal with areas of special stress and therefore of special concern for nursing. Second, we will consider groups of people who are in a state of special stress and need particularly skillful nursing care.

Some areas of the health care facility are routinely involved in far more stressful situations than are other areas of the facility. Such areas include the emergency room, particularly in facilities designated as trauma centers; the outpatient clinic; the coronary care unit; the surgical intensive care unit; and other specialized units, such as burn centers and cancer units. What has been observed, and what I believe is more an *ethical* problem than a managerial one, is that some nurses in these areas cannot function with the degree of calm and inner strength that allows them to be sensitive to the needs of the patients or their families. Some nurses are more concerned about maintaining efficiency and convenience in running the unit than they are about the needs of the family waiting to see a patient in an emergency room or in a coronary unit.

The tragedy of this situation is that it tarnishes the image of the nursing profession, of the health care facility, and, when it is a Christian health care facility, of the entire Christian church. When people are in great need of compassion and understanding and receive only cold, sharp inflexibility, they are hurt and offended. It may take many years and many other loving, compassionate and understanding health care professionals to erase the impression they walk away with at that time.

Areas of special stress are not places for what one author calls "God's grumpy children." Directors of nursing service or others in charge of assigning personnel to sensitive areas, have a moral obligation to make as certain as possible that they are placing the right people in these areas. Furthermore, they need to monitor closely the professional conduct of the nurses in these areas in order to detect problems before they become major disasters. Pastoral personnel are especially concerned about these areas for several reasons. First, having sat with people in these areas, they have learned of their fears, their hurt, and at times their outrage at the way they have been treated. At the same time, they know how difficult people experiencing stress can be and how their behavior presents special problems for nurses and physicians who may be frantically fighting to save lives.

I think some interesting insights can be gained by considering some of the religious-moral aspects of people who are experiencing stress. Some people have extremely bizarre ideas of God. For instance, many people view sickness and tragedy as punishments that have been sent to them by a petulant brat of a God who has been lying in wait to "get them" for their wrong doings. When people who are in a state of genuine stress have these kinds of bizarre attitudes toward religion, they have simultaneous feelings of fear and anger. They need to vent these feelings and, if no one else is around, they often turn their outrage against the nurses, physicians, and the facility.

On the other hand, many people have a more healthy concept of God which gives them an inner strength that can help them in their crisis. However, it takes much time and listening to distinguish between these two classes of people and to respond to the needs or the strengths that are present.

Perhaps the worst mistake one can make is to presume that people who appear calm and in control actually are as they appear. Few people have *really* confronted their own mortality (including clergymen and medical personnel). Consequently, when a person is admitted to a special unit as a patient, nursing and pastoral care personnel should not be lulled by their evidently calm exterior. Sometimes these people are in greater need of compassion and understanding than are those people who wear their emotions "on their sleeves." Often, the latter group calm down more quickly once they become convinced that they are receiving excellent care and that everything is under control.

In situations like those described above, it is certainly desirable to have trained religious health care professionals who can talk to patients or their families. However, this is not always the case, and often the nurse is the person who must respond to the needs of these people. This is one reason why it is important for nurses and physicians to know something of the religious aspects of medical crises. They have to understand that some people experience neurotic guilt, and they must recognize when a person's relationship with God is such that it is counterproductive to his recovery. This does not mean that nurses and physicians must become religious counselors; it does mean that they must realize that religion has a direct bearing on a person's health at this time. Consequently, in certain circumstances, they should call an informed and, if possible, appropriately trained clergyperson to assist the patient in correcting those religious ideas and beliefs that may be causing turmoil or depression.

Another aspect of the study of stress involves people who are in special states of stress, including, among others, persons who attempt suicide, persons who have venereal disease, women who are unwed and pregnant, homosexual persons who hate being such, persons who make sexual advances toward the nurse, persons who are extremely poor or who come from bad home environments, or persons who have entered the hospital as a result of socially unacceptable behavior, such as street fighting, gun shot wounds, stabbings, etc.

These people may not be always pleasant to deal with but the nurse certainly has a moral obligation to render compassionate care to them and to show human concern, even though at times she may be disgusted by their behavior. A nurse is morally obliged to give each patient her professional best. In some of the cases described above, the nonprofessional may not be able to see the illness as such, but a trained nurse certainly should. In fact, the greater the patient's need for sophisticated understanding, the greater the nurse's moral obligation to show that understanding.

In general, patients, such as those described above, need to make some new choices in their lives and reorient their way of living. They may need professional counseling, and all the nurse may be able to do is to start them thinking about seeking further help. The important thing is for the nurse to help them make a decision to do something about their illness. Nurses may find the following counseling model helpful in achieving this objective.

A Model for Decision-Making

1. Get as many facts as possible. Listen for hints of problems other than the one being presented. Often, the first thing the patient mentions is not that which is truly bothering him. It would not be out of place to probe a bit here, as long as one is sensitive to the patient and goes only so far as the patient is ready to go.

2. Identify options: a) What is the present situation? b) What is the patient doing about it? c) What other things can be done? There are usually more than two choices. The more options that can be presented to the patient, the better it is, even though some are obviously unacceptable. It is important to show patients that there are many options and that they are *not* boxed in.

3. Separate those aspects of the patient's situation that can be changed from those that cannot: What is beyond his control, and what is *not* beyond his control? Encourage him to believe in his ability to change that which can be changed. Sometimes the most important thing the nurse can do is to show the patient that she believes in his ability to change. Many people have probably already given up on him or told him that he cannot change his situation, and it will be a tremendous help to him to know that *someone* at last believes in him.

4. Help the patient sort out the underlying issues of the situation, especially the *value* issues. Every option involves a value of some kind, and the nurse should discuss it. Ask the patient to identify the negative and positive consequences of his actions or contemplated actions. Encourage the patient to think through his value commitments. Ask him questions, such as "What do you stand for?" "What do you treasure or really believe in?" "How intensely do you believe in these things for yourself and for others?" Help the patient see that there is no easy or ideal choice. All solutions involve risks and the renunciation of other choices.

5. Help the patient make his own decision in the light of his value system. At times the nurse may disagree with his choice and may tell the patient so, but it still must be his choice. The nurse should emphasize reality, especially if the patient's choice is obviously unrealistic. The nurse must convince the patient that he cannot base his life on an illusion.

50

6. The Christian nurse must be a man or woman of strong principles and values. If the nurse's sense of moral integrity is readily apparent to the patient, that fact alone can be a source of inestimable help and strength to him.

In most cases, if the nurse remembers these six points, she will be able to assist the patient in making those decisions that have to be made if real healing is to take place. This same method can also be used to help a patient make a decision about surgery or some other treatment.

The Nurse

The second major area of concern we must consider is the nurse as a person. Although each of us is unique, there are some personal needs that apply rather generally to all.

The first point I would discuss is the need for the nurse to be an integrated person. She must integrate her own personality, her personal theology, and her professional identity. Each of us must strive to know ourself and our personality for what it is. We all have assets and deficits, and we have all experienced certain growth experiences, various levels of learning, travel, friendships, etc. All of these things are aspects of our personality that we must recognize and accept as our own.

Each of us also has our own theology; that is, theology understood in the strict sense of one's relationship to God. We have different perceptions of God based on different experiences we have had in school, church, and other areas of our lives. As a result, each of us relates to God in our own personal way. For some people, this relationship may be very intense, while for others it may be superficial or nearly nonexistent. Regardless of what the relationship is, sooner or later some patient will directly or indirectly confront us with what we believe. Consequently, we must strive to integrate this part of us with our personality.

Then, too, we have a professional identity. Each person sees herself as a nurse in a particular way. Each has her own concept of what the profession is or should be: What is competent nursing and what is not; who is a good supervisor and who is not; what makes for a superior nurse and what for a mediocre one? I feel that a nurse has a serious obligation to integrate all of this into a whole, because the person who has a fragmented self-image is bound to be an inferior nurse. Therefore, the nurse should be introspective enough to "get herself together," as the popular saying goes. It seems equally obvious that the health care facility has some obligation to provide the means for facilitating such integration. This could be through regular lectures, small encounter groups, interdisciplinary meetings in some areas, or personnel counseling services.

Earlier, we mentioned the need for nurses to be at their best in certain stress areas of the hospital. If one agrees with that premise, he would also have to agree that when a nurse, because of some experience in her personal life, shows signs of becoming cynical, bigoted, or burdened by family cares and concern, the facility has an obligation and the nurse has a right to correct this defect or receive help in solving the personal problems that are hampering her ability to function optimally.

A second point to be discussed in this section is the climate of the health care facility itself. The key word here is *sensitivity*. The climate of the facility refers to more than just cleanliness or a splash of color in the draperies and bedspreads. It refers as well to the kind of atmosphere in which nurses feel that they are respected by their supervisors, that they are trusted as competent individuals, and that their ideas and opinions are given serious consideration.

In terms of the actual physical climate of the facility, the hospital should provide the nurses with slightly more comfortable surroundings in the more stressful areas of the hospital to which they can retreat when they must. Supervisors should be aware of the fact that at times a nurse will be highly affected by the death of a patient even though she was not so affected in a hundred other similar cases.

Certain tasks that nurses perform are extremely stress-provoking. For example, nurses in ICU and CCU units are often forced to make decisions which they do not feel competent to make. In such situations, words of encouragement, support, and understanding are important. In addition, there is a tendency to take for granted really good nurses who have been operating in one area for a fairly long time. When one gets a really good nurse in one of these "high emotion" areas, the temptation is to take him or her for granted. This is a mistake, and supervisors should be careful to determine whether the person is happy to remain in the ward or would like a temporary shift to some other area of the hospital. Sometimes, a few days off or a week or two on another floor is all that is needed to help a highly skilled nurse remain useful in a specialized field. Again, sensitivity is the key. The ability to spot the signs that stress is affecting the nurse is a necessary job requisite for the truly competent director of nurses.

Cooperation between Pastoral Care and Nursing

The third major area of concern to consider is the means by which pastoral care personnel and nurses can work more closely in order to achieve the best treatment for patients and their families. One way to accomplish this is to form a committee made up of a small group of nurses and the chaplain and his assistants. This committee would define the philosophy of care by which both departments will abide.

Unless there is some formalization of ideas and ideals, nothing much is likely to happen.

In addition, it is important to remember that two make a team. Although it is desirable, it is not necessary for physicians and the various therapists and technicians to be involved in some form of "team" meeting to treat patients. If the pastoral people and the nurses are willing to work as a team, they can do so whether or not anyone else wants to be involved. When others see that patient treatment is thus improved, they will get on the bandwagon and participate in discussions of the patients' needs.

The members of the team must respect each other's competence, trust each other as individuals, and be able to mutually draw upon each other's strengths at times. Both nurses and pastoral people will need occasionally to seek counsel, comfort, and compassion from each other.

Summary

To summarize, nurses and pastoral people are morally obligated to be what they profess to be . . . caring individuals. They need to assist and respect each other. Although not all patient cases will require joint efforts, certainly many will and both groups have to be willing to take the time to share pertinent information.

Pastoral care personnel and nurses should sometimes act as "prophets" to one another, in the sense that each will occasionally call upon the other to be their better selves. We all slip at times, and when this occurs, either the nurse or the pastoral person should feel free to challenge his colleague to be more professional, more caring, more concerned. No one has to be or can be another's conscience, but he or she can act as the necessary prod that everyone needs at times. In addition, there must be an atmosphere of mutual support for one another.

Because we live in a pluralistic society, we will sometimes work with persons whose values are quite different from our own. We should respect their opinions and values as far as possible, and we should always affirm their right to hold them. No one has the right to challenge the right of someone with a different value system to work in the facility, unless that person's values clash with the basic philosophy of the department, the facility, or the profession itself. For example, a person who feels that abortion is perfectly acceptable might occasionally work in a Catholic facility. In such a case, the facility would have to insist that publicly, within the hospital, that person uphold the pro-life stance of the facility, even though it may be contrary to his private opinion. If the person's conviction is so strong that this idea is abhorrent to him, then in fairness to his

53

employer and in a sense of integrity to his own conscience, he should seek employment elsewhere.

What we have attempted to do in this paper is to present some pastoral reflections on nursing ethics questions. This is not meant to be a highly scholarly or definitive statement. It is meant to be a means of sparking discussion in the area of cooperation between these two important departments within the health facility. If nurses and pastoral care personnel can come to see that ethics involves more than merely medical decisions, then they can be even more enthusiastic in their efforts to develop and implement a policy of genuine cooperation that benefits not only the patients, but the private and professional lives of the nurses and religious health care professionals as well.

Euthanasia:

Meaning and Challenge

REV. DONALD G. McCARTHY, PhD

There are three areas that I would like to discuss in this chapter. The first is a preliminary general reflection about life-values titled Personalism and Life Control.

The second is euthanasia and the acceptance of death. The acceptance of death is certainly a very traditional concept in Christianity. However, euthanasia is often associated with something a little more vigorous than mere acceptance. Obviously, active euthanasia is associated with the active termination of life or mercy killing. Passive euthanasia, a term that we're hearing more and more in the last five years, refers to a more subtle variation on the verbal phrase; it is not actually an attack on life, but rather a subtle inducing of death.

The third area we will consider represents a follow-up reflection on suffering and death. This reflection will contain some comments about the clinical approach to suffering and death and the way in which it relates to our discussion here.

Personalism and Life Control

I think it is helpful to begin our discussion of life-control in terms of personalism. Within the Christian tradition, there is a long history of the notion of "person," beginning with the earliest discussions about persons of the Trinity and the rather abstract, metaphysical definition of a person as an individual substance of a rational nature. Modern personalism represents a much more dynamic notion of what it is to be a human person. The language of the modern personalists, such as Gabriel Marcel or Martin Buber, is the language of a certain kind of mystery in the development of each person.

The idea of approaching medical ethics and our dilemmas in health care within the context of personalism seems very fundamental to me, if we are working within a faith tradition, because personalism is certainly a part of that faith tradition. The first question that we would ask in terms of person refers to the *value* of a human person.

Is the value of the human person inherent or accidental? Certainly and clearly, a person achieves particular kinds of value as a result of external factors. For example, a person may have treasured friendships that increase his value in the eyes of other people. Notwithstanding, the initial and most fundamental source of value does not come from an appreciation from others but rather from the mysterious inner reality of being a person.

In theistic terms, the personalism of those religions that affirm a personal God attributes dignity to each individual human person insofar as that person is the image of God. In other words, individual dignity derives from some kind of finite sharing in the infinite personhood of God.

We know that to be a human person is to be an individual. The whole biblical tradition of the names that God gives to His people represents an awareness of the unrepeatability of individual persons. In addition, the fact that God knows His people by name indicates an individual kind of relationship. Thus, in the context of religious personalism, to be a human person means to have and enjoy a relationship with God as an individual. It also means that individual persons, because of the gift of the dignity of their nature, can relate to God even prior to the way in which they relate to God as part of a worshipping community. The fact that the value of a person comes from within before it comes from without, namely from the surrounding community, points up an interesting principle.

The fact that existential value precedes functional value raises the question of whether the gift of value can be given already at conception or at a very early stage of gestation. I think that the gift of personhood is given in the earliest stage of existence but needs the environment and, ultimately, human relationships to be expressed.

However, in suggesting that existential value has a more fundamental role to play in our community than functional value, I certainly am not denying that there is functional value. It is part of the human vocation to function and to interrelate. What I am saying at this point is that, if we get down to priorities, the existential value does precede the functional.

One further aspect of this question is the element of meaning. Many questions about euthanasia relate to whether or not the life of a suffering person can really have meaning when the suffering is so extreme and overwhelming during moments of consciousness. There are authors who theorize that when life has no more positive meaning, then the act of terminating the life is not the same as would be the act of murder which would only be taking the innocent life of a person enjoying meaning. So when faced with a situation of intractable pain, we're forced to face this question of meaning.

I don't think that any human person's life ever ultimately loses meaning. It may lose beneficial meaning from the point of view of the experience of that life, and a person experiencing profound pain may say that, in one sense, life has nothing for him but a negative meaning. However, in terms of human life, there is a prior criterion of meaning — the meaning that exists within the gift itself and that meaning is never lost. Thus, we can distinguish between an existential meaning to our lives and a functional or experiential meaning. It is worth noting that the existential meaning to human life does not change regardless of the kind of profound problems that may arise in terms of experiential meaning.

So far, we have discussed life and its meaning within the context of individual persons and of individual persons in relationship to God. Let us now examine the concept of community, the obligation the community has toward the individual. First of all, we must realize that all members of the community share the mysterious gift of being person. The individual gift is given to each individual within a community but through the linking of the community, physical life is experienced as human life. Human experience, then, is an experience that we have in a shared way, with individuals actually relating in and through community.

Thus, there is something in the very essence of being a person which is community-oriented. In other words, persons are by nature community-oriented and cannot be fulfilled outside of community. This, of course, means that just as individuals relate to community so community relates to individuals; consequently, within community there are definite obligations towards individuals.

Two very traditional concepts of community obligation toward individual persons are to foster innocent life and to take reasonable care of life. It is interesting to note that the pagan civilizations that preceded Christianity did not have as firm a commitment to these principles as did Christian civilization. Thus, in terms of commitment to the needs and dignity of the individual, Christianity has helped Western civilization progress.

In any case, the two principles — never to destroy innocent life and to take reasonable care of life — identify two individual rights that are not dependent for fulfillment on age, wealth, size, intelligence, health, genetic pattern, or physical or muscular ability. The rights these principles refer to apply equally to all and are prior to and independent of human function. They are based on human personhood, on existential value, on that mysterious quality of sharing the reflective image of God. Every living person has both a right to life and to reasonable care from others.

The equality principle suggests that we may not destroy innocent persons and that communities are built on the concept of mutual respect. Thus, the sanctity of life principle need not be seen exclusively in a religious context. In fact, there are those who feel that reverence for human life springs from an intuition of the *gift* of being human and being alive and that we need not experience that sanctity uniquely as a religious concept.

With regard to care of life, we are obligated to take reasonable care of human life, not to become fanatics. Maintaining human life is not an absolute goal, since God is the only absolute being and human life is an experience given by God. The death of the body in this life is not an ultimate evil because the person survives. Notwithstanding, we must try to determine guidelines as to what comprises reasonable care. In so doing, we must recognize the right of the patient to participate in deciding whether or not some procedure is going beyond reasonable care.

This concludes my comments on personalism and life value. While I don't pretend that this discussion has solved any of the problems of euthanasia, I hope it has been successful in pulling together the concepts of why the life of any individual is sacred and of what obligations the community has in relation to individuals.

Euthanasia and Accepting Death

The word euthanasia is subject to a number of possible interpretations. Etymologically, it is derived from the Greek *eu* and *thanatos*, meaning a good or peaceful death, and in its earliest use, it denoted merely a peaceful death. It did not specifically mean an organized program to bring about a merciful death, although the traditions of Greece and Rome certainly had set precedents for acts of mercy killing of one kind or another and of individual or assisted suicides.

However, it was not until modern times that the word euthanasia was given the more active connotation of mercy killing, an act deliberately performed in order to accomplish an end of suffering, and, in that sense, an act of kindness performed in order to put someone out of his misery. That has been the meaning of the word in modern times. Thus, the word has come to mean the act of killing for reasons of mercy.

It is possible to find literature that discusses and argues strongly in favor of programs of legalized mercy killing. About 2 years ago, a young man shot and killed his brother who had been paralyzed in a motorcycle accident and who had expressed a strong desire to be put out of his misery. This and similar kinds of cases raise the possibility of some kind of legal acceptance of mercy as a reason for changing the definition of homicide and excusing acts of killing for reasons of mercy. The movement to legalize mercy killing is a real movement, although not a very strong one at this time.

Active Euthanasia

There are two main categories of mercy killing or euthanasia: Voluntary and involuntary. Voluntary euthanasia refers to responding to someone's request and assisting them in their plea for death. Involuntary euthanasia takes place when the suffering person is not or cannot be consulted, and someone else or some other group of persons, such as family or medical committee, decide that this person should be given the benefit of a merciful death. Of course, permitting someone else to make such a decision raises many questions about individual dignity and civil rights.

There are very good arguments against active and direct mercy killing. I will refer to only one source, a classical article by Yale Kamisar which appeared in the *Minnesota Law Review* and which bases its arguments against euthansasia on nonreligious grounds. Kamisar argues that the utilitarian argument in support of euthanasia is not defendable, and that in order to achieve the greatest happiness for the greatest number of people, we must protect life and continue to oppose all acts of termination of life, even in those cases where mercy is the motive. Thus, he argues that the damage to the common good that will result will outweigh whatever individual benefit can be projected by legalizing mercy killing.[1]

When we consider the question of euthanasia in terms of the community, we must ask ourselves if the community at large can justifiably reject an individual by the act of mercy killing. Whether or not euthanasia is requested by the individual, the community (as a community of caring) violates its supportive role when it arranges to eliminate one individual from its context.

Theistic and religious ethicists must further take into account the whole question of stewardship. Are we authorized by God to give up the experience of life through the kind of terminal action euthanasia represents? In a real sense, does not euthanasia represent despair, a rejection of life, along with the suffering that is experienced? If individual persons reject life because of their desire to avoid suffering, are they not, in a very real sense, rejecting God Himself? Certainly, this outlook has been the basis for the strong reluctance within Christian theology, particularly Catholic Christian theology, to accept suicide as morally or rationally acceptable. Rather, our tradition recognizes attempted suicide as an expression of a need, a cry for help. We refuse to accept suicide as a meaningful request that should be authorized within the framework of the caring community. In the same way, we think the caring community should provide alternatives to mercy killing.

"Passive" Euthanasia

The term "passive euthanasia" has been coined in recent years. Unfortunately, it represents a very loose use of language and has the difficulty of being something of an associational term with the broader term "euthanasia." The fact of accepting passive euthanasia would suggest that we should also be able to accept active euthanasia, and, in fact, there are many people who feel there is no real moral difference between the two.

One working definition of passive euthanasia defines it as a means of "inducing a peaceful death by omitting life-prolonging efforts." This definition is inadequate if it is taken in any normative sense. In this context, the word "inducing" is ambiguous, seemingly signifying some middle ground between passively accepting death and overtly performing killing.

In terms of formulating a normative definition of passive euthanasia, a definition which would identify passive euthanasia as a viable option within our traditional ethical framework, some attempt should be made to indicate which life-prolonging efforts are ethically optional. Such an effort raises the whole question of ordinary and extraordinary means of prolonging life, which Father Kosnik already discussed. In talking about ordinary and extraordinary means, we cannot presume that certain means of prolonging life automatically and always fall into either one category or the other. Means cannot be thus conclusively categorized. On the other hand, we must attempt to achieve some kind of objective description of the means of prolonging life; we cannot simply say that the end of a peaceful death justifies any means.

What we are being faced with, then, is the necessity of determining what particular kinds of care are morally obligatory. Such efforts raise the question of omission. I think it is possible to identify omission of ordinary efforts as homicide by omission. In other words, the omission of common and ordinary efforts is the moral equivalent of murder.

On the other hand, the omission of heroic or extraordinary therapy should not be considered homicide by omission. According to the JUCTO theory (Justfiable Use of Conservative Therapy Only) the omission of certain extraordinary efforts should not be considered a legally reprehensible act.[2]

Let us attempt to summarize our discussion thus far. Killing is the act of taking the life of an innocent person, and it is a criminal act of commission. Criminal negligence, which is an act of omission, is still equivalent to killing, at least morally. Although the use of only conservative therapy also implies the omission of certain extraordinary means, this form of omission represents a noncriminal or nonhomicidal omission. In fact, the phrase "justifiable use of

60

conservative therapy only" merely means the justifiable use of medically indicated procedures only. However, the problem still remains of deciding which procedures are medically indicated and which are not.

In attempting to formulate a normative definition of passive euthanasia, we just reject that position which would allow across the board omission of care. Neither can we accept the position that any and all kinds of care must be employed to prolong life. A more acceptable position is that we are morally obligated to provide only a reasonable amount of care.

With malpractice suits flourishing around the country, there are some questions as to whether physicians or hospitals can be guilty of malpractice by omitting what they consider extraordinary means. "Refusal of Treatment" forms signed by patients or their families provide one way in which physicians and hospital personnel can be protected. However, I think that our legal system must seek to clarify on a broader level this whole question of omission of procedures. I think we need to clarify the fact that the omission of fruitless and meaningless life-prolonging efforts (such as those being used in the Karen Quinlan case) is not the omission of due and obligatory life-prolonging procedures. Such an omission does not represent the omission of ordinary care, and is not the moral equivalent of killing. In other words, omission of extraordinary care is not mercy killing but, rather, the responsible practice of medicine. I suggest we avoid calling such omissions by the loose and semantically sloppy term "passive euthanasia."

Suffering and Dying

In discussing suffering and dying, I don't mean to overlook the faith dimension of these realities, but I would like to explore the question of the kind of clinical care available to those who are experiencing intense and unrelieved suffering. Since active euthanasia is often supported as a means of releasing an individual from intense suffering, I think it is advisable to look closely at this whole problem of care for the suffering and dying.

Lord Raglan, who introduced a euthanasia bill in the British House of Lords in 1969, said that he would not have introduced the bill if he had been aware at the time of what institutions known as hospices can do in terms of caring for the dying and for those suffering extreme pain.[3] Just as medieval hospices were guest homes for travelers, modern hospices were also resting places for travelers on a very particular kind of journey — the journey across the threshold into eternal life. Because hospices care for people who are on this particular kind of journey, we might suspect that they are morbid and depressing places. However, the opposite is true. A hospice is not a hospital for dying persons, but a home for living until they die. With the Kubler-Ross type of approach to the reality of the death experience, it is possible to achieve a human community relating to the experience of dying itself.

The numerous British hospices, of which St. Christopher's in London is the best known, will undoubtedly serve as a pattern for the development of similar institutions in the United States. Seven institutions similar to British hospices and conducted by the Hawthorne Dominicans have existed for years in this country. These institutions limit their care to the poor who cannot pay for care, and they accept no fees whatever. They are located in New York City, Hawthorne, NY, Fall River, MA, Philadelphia, Atlanta, St. Paul, and Cleveland.

The two greatest achievements of these institutions and the British hospices are symptom control and spiritual support. Symptom control means primarily pain control. Dr. Richard Lamerton presented a graph in his excellent book, *Care of the Dying*,[4] to show one hospice's achievement in pain control. In the graph the percentages of mild and severe pain-experiencing patients are indicated in three groups, each composed of five hundred admissions. In every group, those who experienced relief in the hospices numbered over 90% and, in the third group, the record was 100% for those with mild pain and 99% for those with severe pain.

Dr. Lamerton argues convincingly that pain can be controlled, and that individual attention to the particular needs and discomfort of each patient is necessary. Both he and other experts in care for the dying are convinced that pain medication must be given on a regular basis so that patients need not fear the onset of a new attack of pain before relief can be given. Lamerton is aware of the fear that dosages will have to be increased to the point where they become useless, but his clinical experience has shown that this can be avoided.

Probably a major reason for the success that hospices have had in controlling pain is the spiritual support they provide. The security of a caring community and the support of family and volunteer staff, together with the promise of immediate and careful attention to pain, offer great psychological strength to the dying patient. Hospices and similar institutions which openly face the reality of death encourage patients to make a spiritual preparation for death and offer strong pastoral care programs. Sister Marie Cordis, administrator of the Fall River home of the Hawthorne Dominicans, was asked about those patients without faith who are dying. She replied, "We just don't see that too often, one who is on his deathbed has an entirely different set of values."[5]

A pilot model hospice for the U.S. is presently under development near New Haven, Connecticut, with the legal title of Hospice, Inc. A building has been designed to care for 44 patients in a setting which serves the unique needs of the dying. All but four of the beds will be in four-bed rooms to create peer support and sharing among the patients and their visitors. Provisions will be made for all day visiting and even for a nursery for children of staff and visitors. Dr. Sylvia Lak who trained at St. Christopher's Hospice in London is medical director of Hospice, Inc.

Although the new building is not yet under construction, a home care program has been operative for two years and has enabled nearly half the patients to die at home. Hospices recognize the advantage patients experience in remaining at home during terminal illness and usually provide outpatient care and home care teams, as well as inpatient facilities. These provisions provide patients with continuity of care and familiarity with the hospice before they ever come there to stay.

Enough has been said here to indicate the importance of hospices in regard to euthanasia. Proponents of euthanasia base their arguments on the desperate situation of some persons who die in intense pain. To kill these patients represents an act of voilence which denies reverence for human life and which corrupts the healing ethos of the medical profession. Instead of taking the "shortcut" solution of euthanasia, responsible health care professionals should choose the alternate solution of hospices and comparable types of care of the dying.

In his book, Dr. Lamerton devotes a whole chapter to the euthanasia debate,[6] arguing convincingly for caring rather than killing. One of the case histories he presents is of a Mr. N., who is dying with a very painful cancer and who is profoundly depressed. His wife had reacted to his illness with anxiety and his three teenage sons with resentment. Mr. N. came to the hospice for care. Subsequently, his wife calmed down. Gradually the boys came to terms with his condition, and began visiting. A reconciliation took place, and Mr. N. eventually died in love and peace. Had Mr. N. been euthanased this could never have happened, and the rejecting family who agreed to the killing would have felt very guilty afterwards. Dr. Lamerton concludes, "If anyone really wants euthanasia, someone must have failed him."[7]

In essence the practice of mercy killing represents a rejection of the suffering person by the human community. Hospices embrace the suffering person with the most meaningful and supportive kind of care, as if the Lord had said, "I was dying, and you comforted me."

Summary

This discussion of the meaning and challenge of euthanasia began with reflections on the dignity and value of human personhood. Those reflections indicate the commonly shared experience of growth and development of persons in community with one another. They also indicate that the value of each person is given to that person directly and individually. The community is called upon to recognize and support that value, in the tradition of the Declaration of Independence which professes that all are created equal and endowed with inalienable rights.

Euthanasia, on the other hand, presumes that human value corresponds to the "meaning" and "function" that persons find in community. Thus when meaning and function seem to disappear, the value of the person disappears and the act of killing becomes justifiable.

Hospices care for the dying in recognition of the inherent dignity of suffering and dying persons, even when they can hardly function in a normal way and find little meaning to life. Through hospices, the human community can affirm its respect for and support of the dying instead of abandoning them.

The art of the healing profession demands the most appropriate kind of care for the needs of persons. When the healing profession can no longer *cure*, it still must *care* for suffering persons. The judgments discussed above in regard to the use of conservative therapy only are inescapable to practitioners of responsible medicine. Hospices practice conservative therapy only, but they still belong to the healing profession.

Stewardship of human life must be both responsible and reverential. Responsible judgments must determine the appropriate kind of cure or care with abiding reverence for the priceless value of every living human person.

FOOTNOTES:

1. "Some Non-Religious Views Against Proposed Mercy-Killing Legislation," *Minnesota Law Review*, Vol. 42 (1958), pp. 969ff. Kamisar's article appears in abridged form in *Euthanasia and the Right to Death*, edited by A. B. Downing, London: Peter Owen Publishers, 1969, pp. 85-133.

2. Donald McCarthy, "Use and Abuse of Cardiopulmonary Resuscitation," *Hospital Progress*, April 1975, pp. 64-68.

3. Richard Lamerton, *Care of the Dying*, Priory Press Ltd., London, 1973, p. 96.

4. *Ibid.*, p. 48.

5. Paul Benzaquin, "Sister to the Dying," *Catholic Digest*, Jan. 1976, p. 74.

6. Lamerton, *op. cit.*, pp. 88-104.

7. *Ibid.*, p. 99.

Nursing as Ministry

LAUREL ARCHER COPP, PhD

In order to understand what we mean when we talk about nursing as ministry, I think we must first attempt to understand the situation of the person to whom the nurse is ministering.

Most hospitalized patients experience a sense of vulnerability in almost all aspects of their mind and body. Often, patients see nurses as the people responsible for intruding or putting something into every body orifice that exists. This intrusion, to which we refer euphemistically as intervention or nursing, involves a tremendous invasion of the body. The necessity of submitting to this intrusion renders the patient's body completely vulnerable. But if the body is vulnerable, how much more so is the mind and spirit. In describing this kind of vulnerability, Louis Evely says:

"What is unbearable is not to suffer but to be afraid of suffering. To endure a precise pain, a definite loss, a hunger from something someone knows, this is possible to bear. And one can live with this pain. But, in fear, there is all the suffering in the world. To dread suffering is to suffer an infinite pain since one supposes it to be unbearable. It is to revolt against the universe. It is to lose one's place in the universe, one's right in it, to become vulnerable over the whole extent of one's being."[1]

Essentially, what we are considering when we talk about this kind of vulnerability is suffering. I particularly want to point out that I am not limiting the meaning of suffering to pain. In fact, in terms of the hospitalized patient, if we think of pain as being stimulus, suffering becomes a response to this stimulus. In considering the nurse's duty to minister, I think we must address ourselves primarily to the question of suffering in response to pain.

First of all, in confronting the patient who is in pain, many nurses insist on a mind/body separation. In effect, they say to the patient, "I am here to care for your physical ills only; therefore, don't ask me to share or understand your feelings and attitudes toward your physical condition and toward the situation in which you find yourself."

In addition, many nurses treat the patient as if his body is a separate entity, completely divorced from his thoughts and feelings.

In the book, *Beyond Endurance,* Walters and Marugg say of this kind of treatment, "Crisp orders, quick responses, their hands busy all about me. They were at my throat, my nose, my limbs, my back, and every touch was torture. They were treating my body as if it were a thing that didn't belong to me — lifting, and clamping, and twisting. At last they said, 'There, she'll do until morning.'"[2]

Many nurses have their own preconceived notions about pain, and these deeply affect the kind of ministering they do. One such idea is that pain follows an hierarchical order, with a gall bladder operation much higher on the pain hierarchy than a tonsillectomy. This is a contrived way of conceptualizing pain, and it does not correspond to the real experience. It is erroneous to compare one diagnosis against another and one patient against another, with the idea that such a comparison will yield a valid pain index. Such validity can be achieved only by comparing various pain experiences of the same person.

In responding to patients in pain, nurses are often so busy telling patients what is going to hurt them that they do not bother to ask patients what it is like to hurt. In my own experience, I found that patients who were undergoing pain so excruciating that there was nothing to do but suffer, actually were doing something else. They were coping. It is in this area of coping that I think ministry really begins, because patients cope with their pain in different ways, and nurses must be aware of these different methods if they are to be able to help.

Some patients cope with pain by responding very actively. Many of these patients can't even stay in bed they hurt so badly. Often, they tend to be "pacers," pacing up and down, up and down hospital corridors. Often, this unabated pacing annoys the nursing staff, and they respond by saying, in effect, "This pain coping mechanism may work for you, but I cannot tolerate it, so please do it someplace where I cannot see you. Better yet, go to bed. I feel better when you're in bed. After all, patients are people who assume horizontal positions, and nurses maintain a vertical stance. So, if you will just lie down, assume a horizontal position, it will be more clear as to what our various roles are and I will feel much better." If the patient persists in his active coping mechanism, the nurse will usually punish him in subtle ways. And, all the time, what he is actually doing is exercising a healthy adaptive mechanism that he could easily do at home but that becomes very difficult to do in the hospital because of prejudices and preconceived ideas about "patienthood."

The second major way of coping with pain is through some kind of mental, as opposed to physical, activity. Many patients recount that they cope with their pain by counting. They count any objects they find — holes in acoustical tile, marks on draperies, tiles on the floor, weaving in the bedspread, etc. Other patients work out math problems. This focusing on details is all-engrossing for the patients involved, and it offers them a vehicle for escaping from their pain or, at least, their preoccupation with it.

Other mental copers are more verbal than mathematical in their focus. Often, these patients verbalize in terms of control words, repeating to themselves over and over, "I won't scream; I won't let it get to me; I can stand this." Very often, by listening to the control words patients use, nurses can determine where the patient is in his suffering. This, of course, is invaluable in terms of ministry.

In addition to control words, patients often verbalize through words of supplication. Old prayers, nursery rhymes, and psalms are popular for this purpose. In the same way, patients will remember a catchy tune, a bit of poetry, or an excerpt from a speech and will repeat these things to themselves over and over. Patients also use derisive words to help them cope with their pain. They say, "This is stupid; this is ridiculous; stop all this." Often, they chastise themselves past the pain. I describe this in "The Spectrum of Suffering."[3]

Some patients don't verbalize at all; rather, they engage in deep thinking and visualization. This can involve many things: Prayer, imagery, concentration, lights and shadows, magnification of sounds, smells, and colors, etc. Some patients construct great, involved schemes in their minds, while others take trips, keeping in mind all details of the proposed route and checking them off as they are passed.

Other patients simply separate their bodies from their minds. Their bodies hurt them so much that they just let them drop away. Still others use counter-pain. For instance, if they are experiencing bad stomach pain, they may rock back and forth, pound their limbs, bite the back of their hand, etc.

What is important for nurses to remember in terms of these coping mechanisms is how best to minister to patients who are engaged in one or more of them. For example, how does the nurse assess what is going on, how does she communicate with the patient about it, and how does she judge the appropriateness of the nursing care and ministry that is being offered? To do these things, it is necessary for the nurse to know the particular meaning that the patient attaches to his pain. Different patients view pain in different ways. They may see it either as a challenge or an enemy, as weakness, punishment, loss, or value.

Patients who see suffering as a challenge regard it as something to be overcome, something with which they must do battle. This concept ties in with the idea of suffering as enemy, as an adversary with whom the patient must struggle. Often patients personify pain and ascribe to it human characteristics. They see pain as treacherous, mean, hateful, detestable, sneaky, intense, obvious, obnoxious, faceless, degrading, cruel, inconsiderate, satanic, nasty, sharp, cunning, nervous, persistent, sly, strong, deceitful, dominating, loud, vulgar, wicked, persevering, testing, tempting, nagging, mysterious, scratching, hoping. Locked into battle with an enemy having these kinds of characteristics, it is easy to understand why patients perceive pain as a challenge to which they respond by coming out fighting.

Many patients view pain as weakness, thinking that if they had been stronger or had led a different kind of life, they could somehow have avoided pain or, at least, gotten through it in a better way. In addition, many perceive pain as punishment, although rarely do they say what they think they are being punished for.

Some people view pain in terms of loss or damage. Many patients have a body concept in which they view themselves as being rather fragile. Any kind of intrusion, any kind of loss of or threat to body integrity, any kind of intervention worries them and makes them doubtful as to whether they will ever be quite the same. I am not referring here to worry caused by losing a part of one's body. I am referring, instead, to the patient's worry that, because of the pain and suffering he has experienced, he will never be the same again. In ministering to this kind of patient, the nurse must keep in mind that the person feels that he has been diminished in some way, that he is less than a whole person, and that he will never again be restored.

Another way in which patients perceive pain is as value. This is not to say that they actively choose to hurt. Rather, they feel that the pain, since it is unavoidable, represents some kind of value. As might be expected, the kind of value that it represents differs with each patient. Some see it as a testing, almost like a coming of age ceremony in which one has to undergo certain experiences before being admitted to the ranks of the initiate. Others see pain as an opportunity to do some necessary soul-searching or as a warning signal that is valuable because it motivates them to seek help.

For others, their own experience of pain gives them insight into the behavior of others who have also undergone the pain experience. Sometimes these other people are relatives or friends whom the patient knows well. In other cases, they are historical figures, such as saints, heroes, and religious personages. I remember one man saying to me, "I never understood why my father hated us so and treated us so badly when we were children. But now I think I understand the reason. He was in pain. Now that I myself have hurt, I can understand how a person just cannot stand to heve the bed jiggled, how he can't stand to have anything intrude on the pain. Everything is a burden."

In responding to pain, patients evidence different feelings. Many fear pain because they fear being abandoned. They feel that it is unpleasant to be around suffering and that if their suffering makes onlookers feel uncomfortable, they will be abandoned by them. From my own experience with the "avoidance" syndrome — the nurse avoids those patients who continue to suffer because they do not reinforce her image of herself as a good and competent nurse — I would say that the patient has every right to his fear of being abandoned. In terms of ministry, the nurse must recognize this tendency to avoid the suffering patient and, instead, help him overcome this fear by demonstrating her willingness to be with him.

Other patients respond to pain in terms of what I call "tropistic yearnings." By this, I am referring to the action of a sunflower turning towards the light. Similarly, in the midst of their pain, many patients yearn for contact with natural things. They say, "If I could just be around the grass and trees and growing things, if I could just be wheeled outdoors and feel the sun on my back, I know I could stand the pain." Unfortunately, very few hospitals and health care facilities provide this kind of opportunity for their patients. In considering this desire for natural things on the part of patients in pain, I wonder about the appropriateness of sending flowers to patients. If the patient needs to align himself with growing things and we send him cut flowers, what else has he to do but wait and watch the flowers die. It is a somewhat bizarre thought.

An essential factor in the whole question of patient vulnerability is the concept of identity. Many patients undergo an identity crisis because they fear that this pain or this surgery will somehow change them, change their identity. Sometimes, the way in which they are treated makes them feel that they are no longer a whole person, but only a body being handled by impersonal "healers." This identity crisis involves cogent questions in terms of nursing ministry: How should nurses respond to it? For instance, should not the nurse at least refer to the patient by his name rather than by his room number and diagnosis ("Mr. Smith" rather than "the gall bladder in 219")? In addition, doesn't the hospital have an obligation to explain his rights to the patient, as well as to explain the procedures which he is to undergo? Can hospitals, ethically, continue to fail to inform patients about issues that directly concern them?

Another area that touches upon nursing as ministry is the area of communication. How does the nurse minister through communication? First of all, she does so by being available. But it is not enough simply for her to be there. In addition, she must listen, answer, explain, repeat, validate, reassure, etc. When asked who the nurse was for him, a patient in pain replied that she was a "translator." In other words, she translated the patient's comments for the doctor, and the doctor's comments for the patient.

For example, suppose a patient, writhing in bed, says to the nurse, "Please, nurse, do something. I've never hurt this bad. I think I'm going to die." Later, when asked by the physician how the patient is doing, the nurse replies, "He seems to be somewhat uncomfortable." Now, that is not what the patient said. In this case, the nurse changed not only the words that the patient used, but the meaning behind them as well. Certainly, this cannot be interpreted as responsible ministry.

As we mentioned above, the nurse also has a responsibility to communicate to the patient what it is that is happening to him. Patients are the only consumers I know of who buy something that the seller refuses to demonstrate or explain. Even when the treatment or the condition is communicated to the patient, the implication of what is being said may not be felt immediately. It may be felt six days or six months later. Since understanding is delayed, ministering may also have to be delayed until the patient feels and, in some way, communicates the need for it.

Patient dependence/independence is another area that calls for a ministry commitment. Nurses often encourage patient dependence simply because it is quicker or easier for a nurse to do something for the patient than to encourage the patient to do it himself. However, nurses must be aware of the fact that robbing a patient of his autonomy can have very serious repercussions.

Although the subject of nursing as ministry is almost boundless in its application, we have attempted to offer some observations on how it operates in the context of the patient in pain, the patient who is experiencing a frightful encounter with vulnerability. It is essential for nurses to remember that the patient entering a hospital and experiencing unaccustomed pain is very frightened. Not only is he doubtful of his identity, but he often feels as if he is being assaulted in those areas of personality that most cogently define who he is. Consequently, in treating this patient, nurses must offer not only physical care but also offer compassionate understanding, if they are to fulfill their responsibility to minister.

FOOTNOTES:

1. Louis Evely, *Suffering*, Herder and Herder, New York City, 1967, p. 152-153.

2. Anne Walters and Jim Marugg, *Beyond Endurance*, Harper Bros., New York City, 1954, p. 3.

3. Laurel Copp, "The Spectrum of Suffering," *American Journal of Nursing*, Vol. 74, No. 3., March 1974, p. 491-495.

Abortion

REV. JOHN F. DEDEK

In the Greco-Roman world in which Christianity arose, abortion was widely practiced, especially among the upper classes, in spite of some opposition from philosophers, physicians, and legislators. Plato had accepted abortion for population control and so had Aristotle, but only before "sensation and life." The gynecologist Soranos of Ephesus (A.D. 98-138) opposed it except when the life of the mother was endangered, and physicians taking the Hippocratic oath swore: "I will not give to a woman an abortifacient pessary." Roman law prohibited giving abortifacient drugs which were dangerous to the mother and forbade any abortion not done with the father's consent. But all the opposition had little practical influence on those who wanted an abortion for personal advantage.

The New Testament, like the Old, contains no clear condemnation of abortion.[1] *Pharmakeia*, the magical practice of medicine by "medicine men," was condemned (Gal. 5:20; Apoc. 9:21, 21:8, 20:15), and this condemnation no doubt included the giving of magical potions and drugs to induce an abortion. But abortion as such is not mentioned in the Bible.

The first clear repudiation of abortion in Christian literature appears in the *Didache*, which was written about 100 A.D.: "You shall not kill. You shall not commit adultery. You shall not corrupt boys. You shall not fornicate. You shall not steal. You shall not make magic. You shall not practice medicine *(Pharmakeia)*. You shall not slay the child by abortions. You shall not kill what is generated. You shall not desire your neighbor's wife."

The word used for abortion here is *phthorion*, which had been expressly distinguished by Soranos from *ekbolion:* it meant "destroying what has been conceived" as distinguished from "expelling what has been conceived."

The *Epistle of Barnabas* (ca. 117-31) put the *Didache's* prohibition of abortion in the context of the command to love one's neighbor:

Reprinted with permission from Sheed & Ward, Inc., New York City. *Contemporary Medical Ethics* by Rev. John F. Dedek, Chapter 7, p. 109-135, 1975.

"You shall love your neighbor more than your own life. You shall not slay the child by abortions. You shall not kill what is generated." And the *Apocalypse of Peter* (ca. 150) says that in the pit of torment are women "who have caused their children to be born untimely and have corrupted the work of God who created them."

Early church fathers like Clement of Alexandria, Minucius Felix, Cyprian, Tertullian, Jerome, Augustine, Basil, and John Chrysostom repeated this general condemnation of abortion. The Council of Ancyra (314) condemned abortion but reduced the penalty for women who aborted an illegitimate child from lifetime excommunication to ten years, and in the years between five hundred and eleven hundred local synods reiterated the canons of Ancyra.

The early Fathers condemned abortion in general and were especially concerned about abortions performed in connection with fornication and adultery. But only Tertullian discussed the problem of therapeutic abortion performed to save the life of the mother. Like the other Fathers he was an antiabortionist, and he defended intrauterine life as fully human: "But for us, to whom murder has been once for all forbidden, it is not permitted to destroy even what has been conceived, while as yet the blood is still being formed into a human being. Interruption of a pregnancy is a hastening of murder, and it makes no difference whether it is a soul already born that is snatched away or a soul in process of being born that is interfered with. He is a human being who will be one; the whole fruit is actually in the seed."[2] But concerning the special case of an abortion that is necessary to save the life of the mother he wrote: "But sometimes by cruel necessity, while yet in the womb, an infant is put to death, when lying awry in the orifice of the womb he impedes parturition, and kills his mother, if he is not to die himself."[3]

In the early Middle Ages theologians and canonists discussed the question of the time of ensoulment: At what point does God infuse the rational soul into the newly conceived body? But the question, originally raised by Jerome and Augustine, was of more speculative than practical interest to them. Even though many believed that ensoulment does not take place until after the body reaches a certain stage of development and that abortion before ensoulment is not homicide, they agreed that abortion before ensoulment is wrong because it has at least the malice of contraception.

Between the 15th and the 18th centuries some theologians began to allow the abortion of a nonanimated fetus to save the life of the mother.[4] Pope Sixtus V in 1588 and Pope Gregory XIV in 1591 condemned contraception and the abortion of animated and nonanimated fetuses.[5] But both popes spoke in general terms about abortion and were directly concerned with the abortions connected with prostitution in Rome. Neither pope mentioned anything about

72

therapeutic abortion, and so their decrees had no influence on the teaching of the more lenient moralists of the time.

The Holy See remained quiet on the matter for another century. Then in 1679 Innocent XI condemned 65 lax moral opinions. Two of these had to do with abortion: (1) it is licit to procure an abortion before the animation of the fetus so that a girl who is discovered pregnant will not be killed or defamed; and (2) it seems probable that every fetus (as long as it is in the uterus) lacks a rational soul and first begins to have one when it is born; and therefore it must be said that no homicide is committed in abortion.[6] These propositions were condemned as "at least scandalous and in practice dangerous."

Contemporary Catholic Teaching

The official contemporary teaching of the Catholic Church took final shape near the end of the 19th and the beginning of the 20th century. One of the principal antagonists was the outstanding moralist of the time, Augustine Lehmkuhl, SJ. One can trace the development of the struggle between him and Rome in the various editions of his *Theologia Moralis.* In the earlier editions he also describes the developing theological scene that brought the Holy See into action.[7]

Many of the earlier authors had defended embryotomy before ensoulment in order to save the life of the mother. Their principal argument was that the fetus was a materially unjust aggressor against the mother's life and that therefore she had the right to defend herself by killing the fetus, just as one has the right to kill a madman attacking him, even though the madman is subjectively innocent and not responsible for his action.

But if the fetus was to be considered an involuntary aggressor, why did these authors restrict embryotomy to the time before ensoulment occurred? Was not the animated fetus also a material aggressor? The reason for their restriction was not that the ensouled fetus was a human being but that he was a human being in the state of original sin and so in need of baptism for his eternal salvation. Hence, the older authors reasoned, the eternal life of the fetus took precedence over the temporal life of the mother. They accepted Thomas's opinion that one may not kill the mother in order to baptize the child, but they did not interpret this to mean that one may not and should not await the death of the mother for the same purpose.

Gradually, however, this strict opinion about the obligation of baptism was displaced, and so was Aristotle's biology.[8] The result was that more recent authors no longer attached any importance to the distinction between an animated and a nonanimated fetus. As far

73

as baptism was concerned, they were content to say that one should try to provide for it insofar as possible, but the mother was not bound to give up her life for that purpose. Hence, Lehmkuhl reports, the modern authors became more consistent: they applied the argument of the materially unjust aggressor to the entire time of fetal life, not just to the earlier stages.

The older authors had described this feticide as indirect killing. They used the category of *indirect* in the same sense as Thomas did when he described the killing of an unjust aggressor: one's direct intention is the preservation of one's own life, and the death of the attacker occurs *per accidens* since it is not the direct object of one's intention.[9] Accordingly, an effect was considered direct or indirect depending on one's intention rather than on the nature or objective thrust of the action. De Lugo and others had resisted this usage, but other authors continued to understand the categories in their Thomistic sense.

A contemporary of Lehmkuhl, Antonius Ballerini, SJ, carefully distinguished the two senses in which various authors were understanding the distinction between direct and indirect killing. Ballerini defended the Thomistic usage. Therefore, he concluded, one may never directly will or intend the death of a fetus, but if the death of the mother and child are imminent, the mother is not bound to die. He argued, as the Salmanticenses had noted, that more than 20 theologians considered the fetus a materially unjust aggressor whose death, as Thomas had shown, would be indrect, not the direct object of intent. This, he said, was also the opinion of Tertullian, and it probably reflected the commonly accepted rule in the early Church.[10]

On November 28, 1872, the Sacred Penitentiary was asked: Is it ever permitted to perform an operation called a craniotomy or a similar operation which per se directly tends to the killing of an infant in the womb? The case proposed noted that the practice was to baptize the infant in the womb before its head was crushed. The Sacred Penitentiary responded that it had given the case mature consideration and that anyone facing this problem should consult the approved authors, both ancient and modern, and then act prudently.[11] Ballerini observed that the Sacred Penitentiary's unwillingness to decide the case was not surprising, since the case was so difficult and learned theologians had defended both sides.

A short time later the archbishop of Lyons asked the Holy See for a decision on a similar case: Is a craniotomy licit when it is the only way to prevent both mother and child from dying? This time the Holy Office was less diffident than the Sacred Penitentiary had been in the preceding decade. On May 28, 1884, the Holy Office replied that after long and serious reflection it had decided that it cannot safely be taught in Catholic schools that a craniotomy is licit even when without it both mother and child will die and with it at least the mother can be saved. And again, prompted by a series of questions from the archbishop of Cambrai, on August 14, 1889, the Holy Office repeated its decision of May 28, 1884, and added that neither can it safely be taught in Catholic schools that it is licit to perform any surgical operation that directly kills either the fetus or the mother.[12]

Immediately after these decisions had been promulgated, Ballerini called attention to the fact that the Holy Office had not made a decision about which of the conflicting theological opinions was true. It had merely said that one of the opinions — the one that affirmed the lawfulness of craniotomies — could not be safely taught in Catholic schools. This meant that it could not be taught with a safe conscience or without danger of error. One must, of course, employ great caution in a question of such gravity as the taking of human life, but one may say that a doctrine cannot be safely taught without judging it to be certainly false. It is enough to judge that it is improbable or only tenuously probable. However, what is improbable at one time, Ballerini pointed out, can become probable or even certain at another.

Lehmkuhl accepted the decision of the Holy Office more gracefully. Even before the action of the Holy See he had considered the more lenient opinion, which permitted therapeutic craniotomies, only a probable one, perhaps even less probable than the stricter one, although still safe to follow in practice. After the Roman decision he admitted that people still could easily be in good faith on this question since the arguments were elusive and the Holy See itself had been in doubt only a few years before. But from that time on Lehmkuhl defended the position of the Holy Office, arguing that it is not easy to see how one can consider the fetus a material aggressor when it is only exercising its natural right to be born. On the contrary, he said, one may say with equal or better reason that the mother is a material aggressor against the life of the child.

Nevertheless, many authors, including Lehmkuhl and Ballerini, pointed out that a craniotomy is one thing and abortion quite another. If one accepts de Lugo's definition of *direct* and *indirect* rather than Thomas's, it is easy to see a craniotomy as a direct attack on the fetus. But it is equally obvious that an abortion need not entail any such direct attack. It is true that when an immature or nonviable fetus is artifically ejected from the uterus it will certainly die. But the mother does not directly attack it. She simply ceases to conserve its life. A mother, these authors argued, is not bound to conserve the life of the fetus at the cost of her own. Her duty to conserve the life of her child, both before and after birth, is limited.

For instance, a mother who is drowning and cannot swim to safety without letting go of her child is not morally obliged to perish with her child in the sea. She may drop the child and swim to safety rather than drown with the baby. In such a situation she does not murder the child, but regretfully permits its unavoidable death.

Therefore, they taught, if without an abortion both mother and child will die, it is better to abort the child and baptize it. One can thus save the temporal life of the mother and better provide for the eternal life of the child. Furthermore, to induce an abortion when the mother's life is seriously threatened is not direct abortion in the theological or moral sense any more than it is direct suicide to relinquish a plank to another after a shipwreck. One can presume that the fetus would renounce any right to remain in the mother's womb in such circumstances, since it would be unreasonable for the child to do otherwise. Remaining in the womb would be useless for the fetus, while by an acceleration of birth its eternal salvation can be better provided for through baptism.

Therefore, they concluded, the principle of double effect has clear application here.[13] The abortion has two equally immediate effects — the saving of the mother and the death of the fetus. One directly intends to save the mother and has a proportionately grave reason for permitting the death of the fetus. The death of the fetus is not the means that saves the mother. It is rather an immediate consequence of the same action that also results in preserving the mother's life.

The Holy Office did not think so. In 1889 the archbishop of Cambrai sent a number of cases to the Holy Office concerning such things as embryotomies, abortions, and the surgical removal of ectopic pregnancies. On August 19 the Holy See replied vaguely, saying that one may not safely teach that it is licit to perform any operation that directly kills either the mother or the fetus.[14] The archbishop of Cambrai then put the question on abortion more directly: If the only way a pregnant woman can save her life is by aborting an immature fetus that will certainly die soon after its removal from the womb, may she permit an abortion to be performed? On July 24, 1895, the Holy Office answered simply and clearly: "Negatively, in accord with the other decrees of May 28, 1884, and August 19, 1889."[15] This reply was confirmed personally by Pope Leo XIII on the next day.

A series of Roman decisions followed. On May 4, 1898, the Holy See decreed that: (1) acceleration of birth is licit for a good reason if the fetus is ordinarily viable; (2) if a woman's pelvis is too constricted for a normal delivery, abortion of a nonviable fetus is illicit, but a Caesarean section may be performed after viability; and (3) an ectopic fetus may be surgically removed if a realistic attempt is made to see that both mother and child will live.[16]

76

On March 20, 1900, a more specific question on ectopic pregnancies was submitted: Is it ever permitted to remove an immature ectopic fetus prior to six months of gestation? On May 5, 1902, the Holy See replied in the negative, since ordinarily a fetus at that stage is not viable.[17] Unlike the reply of 1898, this response lacked the personal papal approbation. Lehmkuhl and Bouscaren continued to argue that in the case of a tubal pregnancy the removal of a part of the Fallopian tube along with the nonviable fetus is an indirect abortion, for this operation, unlike the shelling of the fetus out of the tube, does not directly attack the fetus but removes a pathological tube, with the indirect consequence of fetal death. A large number of moralists have agreed that this operation is morally the same as the removal of a cancerous womb in a pregnant woman and so have approved it as an indirect abortion. This opinion has never been reproved by the Holy See.

In 1917 the new Code of Canon Law reiterated the previous legislation: anyone who successfully procures an abortion is ipso facto excommunicated, and absolution from the peanlty is reserved to the Ordinary of the diocese.

In 1930 Pope Pius XI made a clear summary of the Roman teaching that had emerged and developed during the previous 46 years. In *Casti Connubii* he wrote: "But another very grave crime is to be noted, Venerable Brethren, which regards the taking of the life of the offspring hidden in the mother's womb. . . . As to the 'medical and therapeutic indication' to which, using their own words, we have made reference, Venerable Brethren, however much we may pity the mother whose health and even life is gravely imperiled in the performance of the duty allotted to her by nature, nevertheless what could ever be a sufficient reason for excusing in any way the direct murder of the innocent? This is precisely what we are dealing with here. Whether inflicted upon the mother or upon the child, it is against the precept of God and the law of nature: 'Thou shalt not kill.' The life of each is equally sacred, and no one has the power, not even the public authority, to destroy it. . . . What is asserted in favor of the social and eugenic 'indication' may and must be accepted . . . but to wish to put forward reasons based upon them for the killing of the innocent is unthinkable and contrary to the divine precept promulgated in the words of the Apostle: Evil is not to be done that good may come of it."[18]

During his long pontificate Pope Pius XII repeated frequently in his public addresses the teaching of his predecessor. Speaking to midwives in 1951 he said: "Every human being, even the child in its mother's womb, receives its right to life directly from God, not from its parents, nor from any human society or authority. Therefore, there is no man, no human authority, no science, no 'indication,' whether medical, eugenical, social, economic or moral, that can show or give a valid juridical title for a deliberate and direct disposing of an innocent human life."[19]

The Second Vatican Council made two statements on abortion. In the Pastoral Constitution on the Church in the Modern World (Gaudium et Spes), the bishops said: "Whatever is opposed to life itself, such as any type of murder, genocide, abortion, euthanasia, or willful self-destruction . . . all these things and others of their like are infamies indeed."[20] Near the end of the same document they said: "For God, the Lord of Life, has conferred on men the surpassing ministry of safeguarding life — a ministry which must be fulfilled in a manner which is worthy of man. Therefore from the moment of its conception life must be guarded with the greatest care, while abortion and infanticide are unspeakable crimes."[21]

Finally, in Humanae Vitae Pope Paul VI said: "We must once again declare that the direct interruption of the generative process already begun, and, above all, directly willed and procured abortion, even if for therapeutic reasons, are to be absolutely excluded as licit means of regulating birth."[22] On November 18, 1974, this same doctrine was reaffirmed by the Sacred Congregation for the Doctrine of the faith in its Declaration on Procured Abortion.

Until the 1960s Protestant Christians echoed the ancient Church's condemnation of abortion. Calvin, for instance, described it as an "inexpiable crime." Protestant writers did not engage in the same kind of casuistry as Catholics, but churches, theologians, and preachers of all traditions condemned it in general terms. Bonhoeffer was typical in describing abortion as "nothing but murder."[23]

Karl Barth has also described abortion as murder. Nonetheless he admits that sometimes it may be permitted, in fact commanded, by God as ultima ratio. Exceptions, however, would be rare and limited to situations in which what is at stake is "life against life."[24]

In 1958 the Lambeth Conference affirmed that "the sacredness of life is, in Christian eyes, an absolute which should not be violated." However, it allowed abortion "at the dictate of strict and undeniable medical necessity." Only during the last decade have Protestant Christians generally assumed a more permissive attitude toward induced abortion.

When Does Human Life Begin?

Before turning to the contemporary theological discussion of abortion, it will be useful to consider the nature of fetal life.

In the act of sexual intercourse about 300 million sperm are deposited in the vagina. If an ovum has been released from the ovary, one of the sperm may reach and fertilize it. The ovum will live for about 24 hours; if fertilization does not occur during this period, both ovum and sperm will die. During the first six to eight hours the sperm must be "capacitated" for fertilization by some substance in the uterus or tube. Fertilization usually occurs in the upper part of the Fallopian tube. It is not instantaneous but is a process of taking some minutes. The genes of the father are contained in a packet of 23 chromosomes in the sperm and the genes of the mother in a packet of 23 chromosomes in the ovum. When fertilization occurs these two packets of chromosomes unite to form a brand new genetic package of 46 chromosomes, the normal number in a human cell. This genetic package or genotype, which is absolutely new in the universe, is called the zygote.

After a day or two the zygote, while moving down the tube to the uterus, begins a process of daily cleavage or mitosis, splitting into two cells the first day, four cells the second day, eight cells the third day, and so on. The newly divided individual cells, called blasto-meres, at the end of four or five days form a cluster of cells called the morula.

The morula begins what is called the blastocyst stage. It enters the uterus and starts the process of implantation in the wall of the uterus: one pole of the cluster of cells (the trophoblast) implants itself in the uterus and becomes the placenta; the other pole (the embryoblast) will become the fetus. The trophoblast begins to introduce hormones into the woman's bloodstream to prevent menstruation, which of course would be fatal to the new life. This process of implantation or nidation takes about six days. By the 11th day after fertilization the process is completed.

After two weeks the zygote has become more complex, is about one-tenth of an inch long, and is now called the embryo. It seems that identical twins are formed sometime up to this point by the mass of cells splitting into two separate lots. Perhaps twinning takes place a short time after this. Some embryologists believe that it frequently takes place at the primitive streak stage which occurs at the beginning of the third week. Recombination of split or twinned cells into one individual probably can occur during this same time. Therefore, although a new unique individual genotype is formed at conception, it is not irreversibly an individual until about the beginning of its third week of life.

The embryo stage lasts until the end of the eighth week. The heart begins pumping in the third or fourth week. All the internal organs are present in rudimentary form by the end of the sixth week. Reflex movements occur by the end of the seventh week. At the end of eight weeks the embryo is about one inch long. It is fairly well formed, with fingers and toes recognizable, and electrical activity in the brain can be detected in an EEG reading. After the eighth week it is called a fetus.

Between the eight and twelfth weeks reflex and spontaneous movements occur; the fetus grows to about 3½ inches, and its brain structure is completed. After the twelfth week an abortion by scraping the inside of the uterus (D and C) is dangerous to the mother. If an abortion is performed after this time, it is done by abdominal surgery or by injecting a saline solution which causes an immature vaginal delivery into the amniotic sac.

"Quickening" (perception of fetal movement by the mother) usually occurs before the 16th week. By the 20th week the fetus weighs about one pound and is technically viable. A fetus delivered after 20 weeks has about a 10% chance of survival today, and so its delivery would be classified as premature, not as an abortion. At the end of the 28th week the fetus weighs about two pounds and its chance of survival outside the womb has increased substantially. Practically speaking, it is considered viable from the 28th to the 40th week, when natural birth usually begins.

Those who argue that individual human life begins at the moment of conception find solid support in the teaching of modern genetics. Paul Ramsey says: "Indeed, microgenetics seems to have demonstrated what religion never could; and biological science, to have resolved an ancient theological dispute. The human individual comes into existence first as a minute informational speck, drawn at random from many other minute informational specks his parents possessed out of the common gene pool. This took place at the moment of impregnation. There were, of course, an unimaginable number of combinations of specks on his paternal and maternal chromosomes that did not come to be when they were refused and he began to be. Still (with the single exception of identical twins), no one else in the entire history of the human race has ever had or will ever have exactly the same genotype. Thus it can be said that the individual is whoever he is going to become from the moment of impregnation. Thereafter, his subsequent development may be described as a process of becoming the one he already is. Genetics teaches that we were from the beginning what we essentially still are in every cell and in every human and individual attribute.... What is this but to say that we are all fellow fetuses? That from womb to tomb ours is a nascent life? That we are in essence congeners from the beginning?" [25]

The argument from genotype comes to this. At conception a new and unique genetic package comes into being. This genetic package contains potentially everything that the adult person will become. Man's life is a process of becoming. It would be arbitrary to point to any other moment in this process and say that here a human being emerges. A human being is always emerging, and he is emerging from the initial genetic package which is in potency all that he ever will be.

This position is not only reasonable and scientifically founded; it also most effectively protects the inviolability of human life. For as we shall see, if one tries to designate some point other than conception in human developmental process as the point of inviolability, it is difficult to avoid arbitrariness in assigning that point. If one accepts in principle that a certain degree of development is necessary before inviolability is established, it is possible that the distinction between abortion and infanticide would become blurred and that dangerous discriminations would be made among human beings of varying potentialities.

There are, however, some difficulties that can be raised against this position. For one thing, it gives no weight to the fact that the potentialities in the genotype are conditioned and shaped by its interaction with the environment. A man, the phenotype, is not simply an enlarged or grown-up genotype. One can reasonably argue that a unique human being is not only a product of his genes. He is a product of a genotype in interaction with other things and people. Hominization is a process which is dependent on more than biochemistry, and therefore genetic individuality alone is too narrow a criterion for establishing that one is truly a human being.

What is more, the zygote is not irreversibly an individual until around the end of the second or the beginning of the third week of life. During that time it may split, forming identical twins (or triplets, etc.). And there is evidence that twinned individuals may recombine, forming again a single genotype. The Christian who adopts the position that a human person exists from the moment of conception can explain, of course, that at the moment of twinning God creates another soul for one of the twins and that if recombination takes place, one of the individual human beings dies, even though there is no organic matter that ceases to live. But he must acknowledge that this scientific data considerably weakens his thesis on the beginning of human life. In a footnote to his argument that human life begins at conception, Paul Ramsey admits the point precisely: "The case of identical twins does, however, suggest a significant modification of any 'proof' from genotype. If there is a moment in the development of nascent life subsequent to impregnation and prior to birth (or graduation from Princeton) at which it would be reasonable to believe that an individual human life *begins* to be inviolate, that moment is arguably at the appearance of a 'primitive streak' across the hollow cluster of developing cells that signals the separation of the same genotype into identical twins."[26]

Other moments in the developmental process have also been suggested as the point of inviolability. One rests on the premise that the existence of a functioning human brain is required for the existence of a human person. Electrical activity in the embryo's developing brain does not start until the eighth week, and the cerebral cortex is not fully complexified until around the sixth month of gestation.

If one takes the appearance of electrical activity in the brain of the embryo as signaling its inviolability, then one has a criterion for judging the beginning of human life that is consistent with the now commonly accepted criterion of death. In 1968, when the possibility of heart transplants had made an exact definition of death more urgent, both a statement of the World Medical Association and a report of an ad hoc committee of the Harvard Medical School agreed that death should be defined as an irreversible coma or a permanently nonfunctioning brain. Both documents listed four criteria that signify that a person is no longer alive, even though such vital processes as breathing and blood circulation continue to be artifically maintained. These are: (1) lack of response to external stimuli; (2) no movement or breathing; (3) absence of reflexes, and (4) the confirmatory sign of a flat or isoelectric electroencephalogram (EEG). Therefore, the argument goes, death is a complex process. It consists in irreversible coma or a permanently nonfunctioning brain. A sign of this is a flat EEG. The absence of electrical activity in the brain is evidence that a person is dead, even though other vital processes may be mechanically continued. These vital processes may therefore be terminated for an organ or heart transplant. So, also, at the embryonic stage of life, a flat EEG should be accepted as a sign that an organism is not a living human person but only living tissue. Hence, for a good reason, these vital processes may be terminated.

This argument has a number of obvious weaknesses. One is that the other signs of life, e.g., reflex movements, are present in the embryo. More important is the fact that it is not the comatose state itself but the irreversibility of the coma that is the decisive factor in determining death. The absence of electrical activity in the brain is not permanent or final in the embryo. Just the opposite is true: its potentialities for full human life and personhood set it apart as quite different from a being whose permanently nonfunctioning brain signals that he is dead.

Joseph Donceel, SJ, thinks that in discussing the question of the beginning of human life, we ought to take another look at the Aristotelian-Thomistic thesis of delayed animation or, as he prefers to call it, delayed hominization.[27] Thomas's teaching that the human soul is not created until some time has elapsed in the developmental process of the embryo, he argues, does not have its foundation in outdated biology but in sound philosophy. According to Thomistic hylomorphism, the soul is the substantial form of man. But matter cannot receive its specific form until it is proportioned to it; that is to say, the human body must reach a certain stage of development and complexification before it can receive a human form or soul. The spiritual or rational anima cannot exist except in a highly organized body.

Donceel argues that Thomistic hylomorphism, while probably not defined at the Council of Vienne, always has and still does occupy a favored position in the Catholic church. What is more, delayed hominization is more in accord with modern philosophy's anti-dualistic explanation of man as embodied spirit, as the body of his soul as well as the soul of his body. Donceel concludes: "I feel certain that there is no human person until several weeks (of gestation) have elapsed."

Donceel's arguments have gained the interest and support of other Catholic theologians. Robert Springer, SJ, gives this verdict: "Donceel has uncovered strong historical evidence for his thesis, precedent in official teaching, and theological support to be reckoned with. Join to these his point of the kinship of hylomorphism with modern philosophy and his interpretation of the latest biological findings. It all adds up to a respectable case for delayed hominization. Taking a transtemporal view, we may conclude that the Catholic community enfolds a philosophico-theological pluralism on the question of immediate hominization."[28]

A fair conclusion about the beginning of human life has been expressed by Bernard Häring: "At this present stage of fetology, we cannot state a specific or accurate moment of hominization, although there is never any doubt of the developing process. As the fetus develops, there is an increasing degree of certainty that it has become a human being. On the other hand, there is also a growing consensus that not before implantation, and perhaps not even before the development of the basic brain structure, is individualization a full reality. Therefore, at this stage, there is a higher probability that we are not yet faced with a full human being."[29]

The best answer, therefore, to the question of when human life begins is that one cannot be absolutely sure. The fetus is certainly more than prehuman organic matter. Human life exists at least potentially from the moment of conception. And it is quite likely that it exists from the beginning in the sense of being matter which is activated by a human soul. But there is no way that one can be certain from the evidence available. This, I think, is the only honest conclusion one can draw from the empirical and philosophical data.

Contemporary Theological Opinion

The fundamental premise behind the common Catholic teaching on abortion is that the child in the womb has the same right to life as any other innocent human person. In a public address delivered on

November 26, 1951, Pope Pius XII said: "Innocent human life, in whatsoever condition it is found, is withdrawn, from the very first moment of its existence, from any direct deliberate attack. This is a fundamental right of the human person, which is of general value in the Christian conception of life; hence as valid for the life still hidden within the womb of the mother as for the life already born and developing outside of her; as much opposed to direct abortion as to the direct killing of the child before, during or after its birth. Whatever foundation there may be for the distinction between these various phases of the development of life that is born or still unborn, in profane and ecclesiastical law, all these cases involve a grave and unlawful attack upon the inviolability of human life."[30]

A few weeks earlier (October 29, 1951) he had said: "Now the infant is 'man' even though it be not yet born, to the same degree and through the same title as the mother."[31]

Once it is established as a premise that the life of the unborn child has the same inviolability as that of any innocent person, the conclusions come easily. The fetus may not be killed directly, but only indirectly and for a proportionate reason. Among Catholic theologians there have been some disputes about the application of the principle of double effect to particular cases. They have generally allowed one to remove a pregnant uterus for a proportionate reason, to use other surgical or chemical means to protect the mother even though an abortion may result, and to remove the fetal sac containing a live fetus (but not shell out the fetus) in an ectopic pregnancy. But until very recently they have all agreed that one may never directly destroy or abort a fetus for any reason.

Recently, however, there has been some discontent with this doctrine among Catholic theologians. Bernard Häring has suggested some refinements of Catholic teaching. His opinion is tentative, and he does not recommend its use in practice, since, he says, the presumption is in favor of the official magisterium and a doubt expressed by a theologian does not invalidate the official position. He then suggests two revisions. One concerns the case of therapeutic abortion. He relates the following case reported by a gynecologist: "I was once called upon to perform an operation on a woman in the fourth month of pregnancy, to remove a malign uterine tumor. On the womb there were numerous very thin and fragile varicose veins which bled profusely, and attempts to suture them only aggravated the bleeding. Therefore, in order to save the woman from bleeding to death, I opened the womb and removed the fetus. Thereupon the uterus contracted, the bleeding ceased, and the woman's life was saved. I was proud of what I had achieved, since the uterus of this woman, who was still childless, was undamaged and she could bear other children. But I had to find out later from a noted moralist that although I had indeed acted in good faith, what I had done was, in his eyes, *objectively* wrong. I would have been allowed to remove the bleeding uterus with the fetus itself, he said, but was not permitted to interrupt the pregnancy while leaving the womb intact. This latter, he said, constituted an immoral termination of pregnancy, though done for the purpose of saving the mother, while the other way would have been a lawful direct intention and action to save life. For him preservation of the woman's fertility and thereby, under some circumstances, preservation of the marriage itself, played no decisive role."[32]

Häring argues that the gynecologist acted correctly. The malice of abortion, he says, consists in an attack on the right of the fetus to live. The gynecologist in question did not deprive the fetus of its right to live, because it would not have survived even if he had not terminated the pregnancy. What he did was to serve life as best he could in the situation: he saved the mother's life and preserved her fertility. For Häring, abortion in the moral sense means more than the physical interruption of a pregnancy. It implies that one deprives the fetus of its right to live. But if the fetus has no chance to survive, the fact that the physician causes its biological death a bit early in order to save the mother does no harm to the right of the fetus, since it is not deprived of any personal activity.

Häring's second suggested revision is even more tentative. He simply raises the question about aborting a totally deformed fetus in which there is no development of the central nervous system and brain. He asks if it would be abortion in the moral sense to abort human biological life if there could never be any expression of humanity in it.

Robert Springer, SJ, also has expressed his dissatisfaction with an absolute prohibition of abortion: "The prohibition of direct abortion is an excellent rule, though not unexceptional. He who would attack innocent life must clearly establish his right to do so. The basic question, then, is not: Is it direct or indirect abortion? Rather it is: How great a value must be present to countervail the sacrifice of life?"[33]

Charles Curran takes the same view. In conflict situations where the mother's physical or mental health is endangered by a fetus that will not be able to survive, he suggests that the correct decision cannot be arrived at by considering only the physical act of abortion and its direct and indirect effects. Rather, he suggests, a better solution can be achieved by weighing the values at stake.[34] Specifically, Curran argues that individual human life does not begin until after the possibility of twinning and recombination has passed. After this point an abortion is permissible only if it is necessary "to save the life of the mother or to avert very grave psychological or physical harm to the mother with the realization that this must truly be grave harm that will perdure over some time and not just a temporary depression."[35]

After a long review of the contemporary literature on abortion, Richard McCormick expresses his own thinking on the matter. "Human life, as a basic good and the foundation for the enjoyment of other goods and rights, should be taken only when doing so is the lesser of two evils, all things considered. . . . 'Human life' refers to individual life from conception, or at least from 'the time at or after which it is settled whether there will be one or two or more distinct human individuals' (Ramsey). As this qualifier receives the continued discussion by theologians that it deserves, the benefit of the doubt should ordinarily be given to the fetus. To qualify as the lesser of two evils there is required, among other things, that there be at stake a human life or its moral equivalent. 'Moral equivalent' refers to a good or value that is, in Christian assessment, comparable to life itself. . . . This is the *substance* of the Christian tradition if our best casuistry in other areas (e.g., just warfare) is carefully weighed and sifted; for the permissible exceptions with regard to life-taking (self-defense, just war, capital punishment, indirect killing) are all formulations and concretizations of what is viewed in the situation as the lesser human evil."[36] I believe that McCormick is right in saying that "this position represents an achievement which, in terms of existing evidence, it would be unscientific to deny and uncivilized to abandon."[37]

In summary, therefore, we should say that although the majority of Catholic theologians still support the teaching of the magisterium, which absolutely proscribes all direct abortion no matter what the reason, there is a sizable and growing number of contemporary Catholic theologians who are arguing that there are some exceptions to this general rule.

Although some theologians argue that it is right for the state in a pluralistic society to legalize or decriminalize abortion, no one is supporting abortion for convenience as a moral position. No one is suggesting that abortion is no more than another form of contraception or that the fetus is just tissue in the womb of the mother, merely a part of her body which may be removed for any reason at all.

Contemporary theologians are only returning to an earlier theological position, saying that the prohibition of abortion is not an absolute one. Ordinarily the purposeful destruction of the fetus is morally wrong. But exceptions to this rule have to be made when a proportionate value, another life or its moral equivalent, is at stake.

Assisting at Abortions

The legalizing of abortion has given rise to a new problem of conscience for some Catholic nurses, interns, and paramedical personnel working in public and non-Catholic health facilities. Should they cooperate in any way with the abortions that now are being performed in the hospitals and clinics in which they are working?

Those in charge of these health facilities are rightly concerned that every abortion be performed with maximum medical safety for the pregnant woman. Therefore, after the abortion they generally require the woman to stay for a time in a recovery room, where she will be kept under observation for possible postoperative complications such as abscess, hemorrhage, and so on. Such complications are unusual, but if they do develop they can present a severe threat to the woman's life, and in that event, immediate attention by trained personnel is critically important.

Preoperative care is also important. Before the abortion an intern interviews and examines the woman to learn about any other diseases she may have, to check her blood pressure, heart, lungs, and so forth, so that if any complications occur after the operation an accurate diagnosis can be promptly made. A surgical nurse is even more directly involved. Her job may be to set out the instruments, hand them to the doctor, and so on.

In some rare instances administrative policy has required interns, nurses, and paramedics to perform these services — if they refused, they were fired or asked to resign. But even in the past such cases were unusual. At the present time hospital personnel are generally given a free choice. If they ask to be excused from this work for reasons of conscience, the administration will honor their request and there will be no recrimination. In some places discriminatory hiring practices have shown up, and sometimes the official administrative policy is compromised by subtle pressures or punishment by the particular individuals in charge. But in most cases the official policy is carried out in practice as meticulously and fairly as possible.

This is the context in which the moral question arises. What is the moral responsibility of those who believe that abortion is immoral? Should they participate in any way or should they ask to be excused for reasons of conscience?

In themselves preoperative and postoperative care are morally good. It is the abortion that is immoral, not the medical care for the health and safety of the woman. This is exactly the same kind of care that an intern or nurse would give at a perfectly moral operation. The problem is that here it is not given at a perfectly moral operation. It is given in connection with an abortion.

If it is given with internal approval of the abortion, it is what theologians call formal cooperation, which is never permissible precisely because of one's internal approval of an immoral act. The formal cooperator is an accomplice who personally intends and wills not only the preoperative and postoperative care but the abortion as well. He shares in the blame for the abortion because of his bad will.

But it is quite possible for someone to give preoperative and postoperative care without approving of the abortion. Such care given without internal approval of the abortion is not formal cooperation. Rather it is called material cooperation. Material cooperation is permissible only if one manifests his disapproval so as to prevent scandal and at the same time has a proportionately serious reason for cooperating.

Therefore, the difficult decision of conscience revolves around this question: Do I have a proportionately serious reason for materially cooperating in an abortion? It is obvious at once that no universal answer can be given. The correct decision will depend on a complex of competing values in the particular situation. However, some broad statements can be made to illustrate how Catholic moral theologians generally evaluate the issue.

Practically all theologians agree that material cooperation in an abortion would be justified if the intern or nurse were threatened with some serious harm, for example, losing one's position with considerable personal loss. Also, many theologians argue that even if Catholic interns or nurses could get equally good or even better positions elsewhere, it does not follow necessarily that they should resign their positions at state institutions, since the spiritual and moral good they can do there may easily compensate for their occasional material assistance at an abortion.

In the present situation, however, loss of job is seldom, if ever, an issue. Generally speaking, no one's job is on the line. In most health facilities individual decisions of conscience will be respected without recrimination. And, normally, no serious harm will be caused to anyone if Catholic nurses and interns ask to be excused from assisting at abortions. What this means is that, ordinarily, there will be no proportionate reason to justify their material cooperation in abortions.

Therefore, as a normal rule in the present circumstance, Catholic nurses, interns, and paramedics should ask to be excused for reasons of personal conscience from assisting at abortions in any way. Preoperative and postoperative care can easily be given by others who have no conscientious objections to abortion.

This rule, of course, is not absolute. Certainly there will be exceptions to it. Emergency situations may develop in which a Catholic would be morally obliged to give postoperative care to a woman in need of it. And there may be other considerations of good to be accomplished or harm to be avoided which in a particular situation would justify material assistance.

But in the absence of such serious reasons, a Catholic should abstain from any assistance directly connected with abortions. Although abortion is no longer a crime, it is still a sin. It is not enough for a Catholic merely to believe this internally. He should give visible witness to his convictions.

Hopefully, this common witness will say something to the medical profession and perhaps help sensitize others to the value of human life, whereas failure to give practical testimony could be scandalous in that it would tend to confirm the convictions of those who place less value on the lives of unborn children.[38]

FOOTNOTES:

1. Exodus 21:22 requires that a man pay an appropriate fine if he accidentally causes a woman to have a miscarriage.

2. *Apologeticus* 9, 8.

3. *De Anima* 25, 4.

4. Cf. John F. Dedek, *Human Life* (New York: Sheed and Ward, 1972), pp. 38-40.

5. *Ibid.*, pp. 41-42.

6. DS 2134-2135.

7. See ed. 7, vol. 2, tract. 2, cap. 3, n. 839-849.

8. In 1869 Pius IX dropped the distinction between an animated and nonamimated fetus in his reorganization of canon law.

9. *Summa theologae* II-II, 64, 7.

10. Antonius Ballerini, SJ, *Opus Theologicum* Morale, vol. 2, tract. 4, sect. 5, cap. 1, dub. 4; and *Compendium Theologiae Moralis*, Tom. I, tract. de Praecepto 5 Decalogi, cap. 2, art. 3.

11. Quoted in Lehmkuhl and Ballerini.

12. Quoted in Lehmkuhl and Ballerini.

13. The principle of double effect is generally enunciated something like this: it is morally permissible to place an action which has two foreseen effects, one good and one bad, if four conditions are all verified: (1) the action itself is good or indifferent; (2) the good effect is not produced by means of the bad effect; (3) only the good effect and not the bad effect is directly intended; (4) there is a proportionate reason for placing the action and permitting the bad effect.

The *first condition* requires that the action itself be good or at least indifferent. The reason for this requirement is that if the action is morally wrong in itself, then it is already illicit independent of its consequences.

The *second condition* requires that the good effect be not produced by means of the bad effect. The reason for this is that we may not do evil that good may come of it (Rom. 3:8). For to will evil as a means is to will it in itself if not for itself, and to deliberately will evil is morally wrong.

To understand the implications of this second condition one should notice that the good and the evil effects can be related in three ways: (1) the action primarily produces the evil effect and the evil effect produces the good effect (example: a man in a burning building puts a loaded shotgun in his mouth and pulls the trigger so that he will avoid the pain of burning to death); (2) the action primarily produces the good effect and the good effect produces the bad effect (example: a surgeon saves the life of a despotic dictator and as a result his despotic rule continues); (3) the action produces both effects together and independently of each other (example: an aviator drops a bomb on a ship killing both combatants and innocent passengers). What is implied in this second condition is that numbers 2 and 3 can be licit but number 1 cannot.

It is important to notice that the relation between the two effects that is relevant here is the relation of causality, not merely that of time. Temporal priority usually indicates a casual connection, but this is not necessarily the case. (Example: a surgeon removes a cancerous uterus containing a live, nonviable fetus. In order to remove the uterus he must first cut veins and arteries, thereby killing the fetus by severing its only lifelines. The death blow is first administered to the fetus chronologically before the womb is removed, and as a matter of fact the fetus is usually, though not always, dead before the uterus has been removed. Nonetheless, the same sealing of veins and arteries would be necessary even if there were no fetus present. Both effects issue from this act equi-immediately in the order of causality.) It is important to notice that the fact that the evil effect will certainly follow does not mean that it is the means to the good effect. (Example: the death of the fetus, although certain, is not the means to the mother's cure, but simply an inevitable effect of the hysterectomy.)

The *third condition* demands that only the good effect and not the evil effect be directly intended as the end of the action. For if evil is the end, the will embraces evil; that is to say, it deliberately chooses it.

The *fourth condition* is that there be a proportionate reason for placing the cause and permitting the evil effect. A proportionate reason is required to permit the foreseen evil because we are obliged not only not to intend or do evil, but also to avoid it insofar as it is morally possible to do so. A proportionate reason is sufficient to permit evil because if there is a proportionate reason, the avoidance of the evil is judged to be morally impossible and we are excused from the general obligation to avoid evil; that is to say, it is then reasonable to place the good act even though it has an unavoidable bad consequence.

14. DS 3258.

15. DS 3298.

16. DS 3336-3338.

17. Quoted in Lehmkuhl.

18. Paulist translation, n. 63-66.

19. Pius XII, AAS 43 (1951) 838-839.

20. *Gaudium et Spes*, n. 27.

21. *Ibid.*, n. 51.

22. Paul VI, *Humanae Vitae*, 14.

23. Dietrich Bonhoeffer, *Ethics* (New York: Macmillan, 1965), p. 176.

24. Karl Barth, *Church Dogmatics*, vo. 3, part 4, p. 55.

25. Paul Ramsey, "The Morality of Abortion," in Daniel H. Labby, ed., *Life or Death: Ethics and Options* (Seattle: University of Washington Press, 1968), pp. 61-63.

26. *Ibid.*, p. 63, no. 1.

27. Joseph Donceel, SJ, "Animation and Hominization," *Theological Studies* 31 (1970): 76-105.

28. Robert Springer, SJ, "Notes on Moral Theology," *Theological Studies* 31 (1970): 500-501.

29. Bernard Häring, *Medical Ethics* (Notre Dame: Fides, 1973), p. 101.

30. AAS (1951) 857.

31. AAS (1951) 838.

32. Bernard Häring, "A Theological Evaluation," in John T. Noonan, Jr., ed., *The Morality of Abortion* (Cambridge: Harvard University Press, 1970), pp. 136-137.

33. *Theological Studies* 31 (1970): 493.

34. Charles Curran, *Contemporary Problems in Moral Theology* (Notre Dame: Fides, 1970), pp. 144-145.

35. Charles Curran, *New Perspectives in Moral Theology* (Notre Dame: Fides, 1974), p. 191.

36. Richard McCormick, SJ, "Notes on Moral Theology," *Theological Studies* 35 (1974): 354.

37. *Ibid.*

38. Cf. ad hoc Committee on Pro Life Activities, National Conference of Catholic Bishops, "Pastoral Guidelines for the Catholic Hospital and Catholic Health Care Personnel," (Washington, D C: United States Catholic Conference, 1973).

Affirming Human Life

KEVIN O'ROURKE, OP, JCD

Two years ago, while giving a talk to administrators of nursing homes and long-term care centers, I evaluated the Living Will as put forth by the Euthanasia Educational Council and gave my reasons for opposing this document. After I had finished my presentation, one of the administrators said, "We think that your reasoning is logical and that there is some basis for your position, but, as a matter of fact, people still wish to sign documents of this nature." Others attending the meeting agreed with this statement.

Because I think that those who profess Christianity must try to transform rather than merely criticize the secular, I volunteered to write such a document. With the help of other people at The Catholic Hospital Association, a document was written and later approved by the CHA Board of Directors. In less than two years, over 1,000,000 copies of this document, the Christian Affirmation of Life (CAL), have been distributed. In this chapter, I would like to again present briefly my evaluation of the Living Will, demonstrate how the Christian Affirmation of Life differs from it, and then offer some suggestions for using the latter document.

As you know, the Living Will states briefly:

"If there is no reasonable expectation of my recovery from physical or mental disability, I request that I be allowed to die and not be kept alive by artificial or heroic measures.... I ask that medication be mercifully administered to me for terminal suffering even if it hastens the moment of death. ... I am not asking that my life be directly taken, but that my dying be not unreasonably prolonged."

If we interpret the words "artificial and heroic measures" to mean the same thing as "extraordinary means," it is clear that the Living Will does not contradict traditional Christian teaching. The validity of this interpretation is borne out by the respect for life displayed in this statement of the Living Will, "I am not asking that my life be directly taken, but that my dying be not unreasonably prolonged." Christian teaching requires that a person use ordinary means to prolong life, but allows one to refuse means which are judged to be extraordinary.

92

Moreover, if the primary purpose of a certain medication is to alleviate pain, traditionally Christians have held that pain-relieving medication can be administered to a dying person, even though the indirect effect might be to hasten death. Allowing a person to die when death is inevitable, or even indirectly hastening death when trying to relieve pain, are not contrary to the traditional Christian manner of caring for the terminally ill. Hence, the statements of the Living Will are not in basic conflict with Christian tradition.

Since the Living Will is signed well before one is terminally ill, it prompts people to face death before it becomes imminent. Psychologically and spiritually, this confrontation is beneficial; confronting death and discussing it in a realistic manner when death is not imminent will help people accept death more readily when it comes. The Living Will also lessens the possibility of useless, painful, and expensive medical treatment as death approaches. Perhaps this is its strongest appeal.

At present, the Living Will is not accepted as a legal and binding document in any state of the Union, but bills to have it recognized as a law have been introduced in many states, and proponents of the document seek to have it legalized as a contract. If the Living Will becomes law, physicians and families of those who are terminally ill would be required under penalty of law to follow the stipulations of the document. If such an eventuality would occur, how would we then evaluate the Living Will?

In spite of the fact that the Living Will is not contrary to traditional Christian teaching in its basic statement, and in spite of the fact that it does help people prepare for death, I believe that it has several drawbacks.

First of all, because it rejects the use of *all* "artificial or heroic means" it implies that decisions concerning which means to use to prolong life when a person is in danger of death can be made in an abstract or impersonal manner. Decisions as to what constitutes proper care (and traditionally we use the terms "ordinary" and "extraordinary" means) can be made only in terms of each particular case and each particular person who is dying. We cannot specify that the use of a particular medical treatment or machine or surgical technique is always either ordinary or extraordinary; we must first examine the situation at hand. We must consider the person and what that person is undergoing, what capabilities that person has for life, and even whether that person will be able to finance the technique or surgical procedure in question.

For example, most people consider penicillin an ordinary means of prolonging life. It is plentiful and fairly economical. But, for the person who is violently reactive or allergic to penicillin, would penicillin be an ordinary means? Not at all. Again, is putting a person on a respirator an ordinary means of prolonging life? If the respirator were to be used only for a few days, perhaps it would be. However, would it be considered an ordinary means if the person would have to be on it for 20 or 30 years? We cannot make judgments about particular cases unless we know the facts and the circumstances involved.

Pope Pius XII, who is quoted not only by Catholics but also by non-Catholics in regard to this matter, stated: "When making a decision about ordinary or extraordinary means, one must consider whether the means in question involve any grave burden for oneself or for another according to the circumstances of person, place, times, and culture." *(The Pope Speaks,* Vol. 4, #4, 1958)

If legislatures were to give the Living Will the force of law, then the sensitive decisions concerning ordinary and extraordinary means and reasonable expectation of recovery would be made by legislators, judges, and juries in an *apriori* and legalistic manner, rather than by the patient, the physician, or the family, with the good of the particular patient in mind. Moreover, if the decision concerning ordinary and extraordinary means becomes mechanical or legalistic, physicians are liable to give up efforts that might restore life. Deciding when a particular procedure will benefit a patient is often a difficult task. Hence, the physician should be given the freedom to make his decision without worrying about legalisms or malpractice suits.

The Christian Affirmation of Life (CAL) seeks to insure that the decision concerning ordinary and extraordinary means will be made in a careful and personal manner. First of all, the Affirmation is not presented as a legal document, but rather as a document of reflection and meditation. Any move to make the provisions of the Affirmation legally binding would be opposed strenuously. As pointed out in The Karen Quinlan Decision, courts would have an impossible time enforcing such documents.

Secondly, the stipulations of the document are phrased in such a way that the wishes of the patient, should he not be able to express his own desires, do not preempt the judgment of the family and the physician. The Affirmation states:

"I request that I be informed as death approaches . . . and I request that, if possible, I be consulted concerning the medical procedures which might be used to prolong my life as death approaches. If I can no longer take part in decisions concerning my own future and there is no reasonable expectation of my recovery from physical and mental disability, I request that no extraordinary means be used to prolong my life."

Thus, the Affirmation does not seek to determine what constitutes ordinary and extraordinary means for the person in question. Rather, it implies that, if a person is unable to be consulted, the family and

CHRISTIAN AFFIRMATION OF LIFE

Because of my belief:

I, _____
request that I be informed as death approaches so that I may continue to prepare for the full encounter with Christ through the help of the sacraments and the consolation and prayers of my family and friends.

I request that, if possible, I be consulted concerning the medical procedures which might be used to prolong my life as death approaches. If I can no longer take part in decisions concerning my own future and there is no reasonable expectation of my recovery from physical and mental disability, I request that no extraordinary means be used to prolong my life.

I request, though I wish to join my suffering to the suffering of Jesus so I may be united fully with him in the act of death-resurrection, that my pain, if unbearable, be alleviated. However, no means should be used with the intention of shortening my life.

I request, because I am a sinner and in need of reconciliation and because my faith, hope, and love may not overcome all fear and doubt, that my family, friends, and the whole Christian community join me in prayer and mortification as I prepare for the great personal act of dying.

Finally, I request that after my death, my family, my friends, and the whole Christian community pray for me, and rejoice with me because of the mercy and love of the Trinity, with whom I hope to be united for all eternity.

Signed _____

Date _____

physician should decide as to what they consider ordinary and extraordinary care. The Affirmation merely requests that if, after due consideration, a particular means is considered extraordinary, it not be utilized if there is no reasonable hope of recovery. In other words, when a person signs a Christian Affirmation of Life, he asks that his family and physician act in a Christian manner if he is near death and there is no hope of his recovery. This request should be merely one factor, perhsps not the determining factor, in a number of factors that must be weighed before a mature decision of conscience can be reached.

A second shortcoming of the Living Will is perhaps more subtle, but nonetheless serious. This is the *atmosphere* that it creates. The Living Will seems to say, "How little can we do for the dying person," rather than "How can we best care for the dying person," which is the real question a Christian faces when someone is suffering from terminal illness. Many of the articles written in favor of the Living Will merely emphasize the expense of keeping the elderly alive, without referring to the contributions that they have made and are making to society at the present time.

Furthermore, the Living Will does not refer to love, hope, life after death, responsibility to God as Lord and Creator, the life of our Savior, Jesus Christ, or the value of suffering for us. Removing death from the context of love, life, and salvation makes it a meaningless, dismal, and fear-filled event. Every person who is contemplating his own death and the kind of treatment he would want to receive is not really receiving full pastoral consideration unless the realities of the Holy Spirit, the creative love of God, and the redeeming act of Christ are introduced into the context of the decisions being made.

The Christian Affirmation of Life also attempts to emphasize, in this context of life and death, the presence of fear, suffering, sorrow and sin, need for reconciliation, the help that other Christians can offer through prayer and mortification, and the role of sacramental participation in the process of dying. Although this list is rather lengthy, death is one of the greatest human mysteries and should be contemplated and experienced in conjunction with the other mysteries God has given us, particularly the mystery of His own love and the mystery of our redemption.

Perhaps some of the shortcomings of the Living Will that I have mentioned (namely, the fact that it creats a rather fear-filled atmosphere and the fact that it impersonalizes the decision about ordinary and extraordinary means) do not seem too serious. However, its third shortcoming is even more dangerous, for the efforts being made to make people accept the Living Will and to make its stipulations enforceable by civil law appear to be a step forward in the drive to legalize active euthanasia of the retarded, elderly, and infirm. As Dr. Joseph Fletcher points out, the Euthanasia Educational Council, which publishes the Living Will, is a nonprofit arm of the Euthanasia Society of America. The parent society was founded to foster direct or active euthanasia.

Many of the most active sponsors of the Living Will are also active proponents of abortion on demand and direct euthanasia. Apparently, it is a small step from mandatory withholding of care to legalizing the direct taking of innocent life. One of the first people in the U.S. to introduce a bill to legalize passive euthanasia was a Florida physician, Dr. Walter Sackett, a member of his state legislature. In testifying before the Special Committee on Aging of the U.S. Senate about his bill to legalize passive euthanasia, he made it clear that he wanted this bill passed in order to save money that would otherwise be spent on caring for retarded or invalid people and to use it, instead, for other medical purposes. In other words, he moved beyond passive to active euthanasia.

Morally speaking, allowing people to die when death is imminent and eliminating severely retarded people for financial reasons are as different as night and day, but Dr. Sackett put the two in the same category. If passive euthanasia is enacted as statute of law and becomes mandatory, I wonder whether active euthanasia wouldn't be far behind.

The danger connected with any law which would make withholding care mandatory was expressed aptly by another person who testified before the Senate's Special Committee on Aging. Dr. Elizabeth Kubler-Ross declared: "I am against the legalization of any such bills which allow passive euthanasia, because their loopholes will allow the elimination of those lives that are too costly or too much of a burden."

In order to avoid any connection with active euthanasia or elimination of the retarded, infirm, or senile, the Christian Affirmation of Life stresses the love that the Creator has for each person. Moreover, the Affirmation declares that the dignity and worth of each individual person is founded upon the relationship of love in Christ that God has for each person, and not upon the usefulness or the effectiveness of any individual person in society. Hence, the Christian Affirmation of Life explicitly rejects the "quality of life" ethic that would determine which people live and which people die. If we allow the court or legislatures to determine what is meaningful life, as the decision of the Supreme Court on abortion indicates they might do, we are going to live in an increasingly barbaric and brutal society.

Anything we do in regard to people who are dying, weak, or ill should be seen within a total Christian context. Are we exercising mercy, care, and love? Or are we simply, for pragmatic reasons, serving our own needs and desires under the guise of mercy, care, and love? In this society at this particular time, we must continually remind ourselves that violence is self-destructive. Once we allow violence to enter, we are in danger not only of destroying ourselves but our whole common life in society as well.

When we base the radical worth and dignity of any person upon a quality of life ethic, we open the door to wanton killing of anyone who can be declared less than normal from some point of view. When the Supreme Court determined that only those with "meaningful life" have the right to protection under the 9th and 14th amendments, it opened the door to innumerable atrocities under the cover of "mercy." Not only will unborn human beings be sacrificed because of the quality of life ethic, but also those born human beings who do not lead a life that can be judged meaningful by someone or some committee.

Lastly, how should the Christian Affirmation of Life be used? The first use would be to meet the need which brought the Affirmation into being, namely for people who wish to make some statement concerning the type of treatment they desire if they are near death and unable to speak for themselves. Even though I have criticized the Living Will rather severely, I do not repudiate completely the concept of a document that expresses this type of desire. Some people have questioned the propriety of the Affirmation of Life, declaring that Christians should have nothing to do with a document that concerns itself with the care rendered at the time of death. However, the fact that many people have expressed an interest in a document such as the Living Will shows that a need exists, and Christians should respond to that need. We should provide these people with a means of fulfilling their desire to avoid unnecessary, expensive, or even painful treatment at the time of death.

The second and perhaps even more worthwhile use of the CAL is to help people understand suffering, dying, and death in a total faith context — to understand these realities in relationship to other aspects of faith. For example, some college and high school teachers have used the Affirmation as a framework for discussing a Christian view of death and dying with their students. Similarly, many hospital chaplains use it to "break the ice" and to initiate conversations concerning issues which are sometimes difficult to approach but which are nonetheless very sensitive and important to each individual person.

The main complaints about the CAL have come from physicians who maintain that it gives the impression that all doctors try to keep every patient alive as long as is humanly possible. This, of course, is not the purpose of the CAL. However, in this regard, it is worthwhile to consider the words of Dr. Frank Ayd, writing in his January, 1975 *Medical-Moral Newsletter:*

"This editor has stated repeatedly that there is no doubt that there would be less pressure for euthanasia, if physicians did not use all the resources at their command to delay death in every patient. There should be no need for euthanasia and there would be no demand for it or for suicide education, if doctors acknowledge that it is neither scientific nor humane to use artificial life-sustainers when death is imminent and inevitable and realistic hope of recovery has evaporated. Also there should be no need or demand for euthansaia or suicide education, if physicians unhesitatingly administer whatever amount of pain-relieving drugs a dying patient needs. The medical profession has the power to erase any demand for legalized euthanasia or for suicide education. All physicians have to do is apply their skills prudently as they are morally and legally empowered to do." *(Medical-Moral Newsletter,* Jan. 1975, Vol. XII, #1, St. Anthony Messenger Press, Cincinnati, Ohio)

Whether or not we agree with Dr. Ayd's statement is not the point. Rather, the point is that his statement indicates that there are situations which justify such things as the Christian Affirmation of Life. In some situations, both patients and families suffer because life is prolonged for too long a time.

The Christian Affirmation of Life is not intended to be a substitute for or a contradiction of the Living Will. Rather, it seeks to transcend the Living Will, overcoming some of its defects and presenting its thought according to a faith-dominated vision. To discuss objectively something with which one has been intimately involved for some time is not easy. Since I have been involved in the Affirmation of Life from its inception, I imagine that some of you will have certain reservations about some of my statements. Nevertheless, I would like to conclude with one thought I hope everyone can accept without hesitation: Namely, read the Christian Affirmation of Life carefully, because the life you affirm may be your own.